Craniosynostosis: Current Perspectives

Editor

SRINIVAS M. SUSARLA

ORAL AND MAXILLOFACIAL SURGERY CLINICS OF NORTH AMERICA

www.oralmaxsurgery.theclinics.com

Consulting Editor
RUI P. FERNANDES

August 2022 • Volume 34 • Number 3

ELSEVIER

1600 John F. Kennedy Boulevard • Suite 1800 • Philadelphia, Pennsylvania, 19103-2899

http://www.oralmaxsurgery.theclinics.com

ORAL AND MAXILLOFACIAL SURGERY CLINICS OF NORTH AMERICA Volume 34, Number 3
August 2022 ISSN 1042-3699, ISBN-13: 978-0-323-92002-5

Editor: John Vassallo; j.vassallo@elsevier.com
Developmental Editor: Jessica Nicole B. Cañaberal

Oral and Maxillofacial Surgery Clinics of North America (ISSN 1042-3699) is published quarterly by Elsevier Inc., 360 Park Avenue South, New York, NY 10010-1710. Months of issue are February, May, August, and November. Business and Editorial Offices: 1600 John F. Kennedy Blvd., Suite 1800, Philadelphia, PA 19103-2899. Periodicals postage paid at New York, NY and additional mailing offices. Subscription prices are $405.00 per year for US individuals, $961.00 per year for US institutions, $100.00 per year for US students/residents, $478.00 per year for Canadian individuals, $990.00 per year for Canadian institutions, $100.00 per year for Canadian students/residents, $530.00 per year for international individuals, $990.00 per year for international institutions and $235.00 per year for international students/residents. To receive student/resident rate, orders must be accompanied by name or affiliated institution, date of term, and the *signature* of program/residency coordinator on institution letterhead. Orders will be billed at individual rate until proof of status is received. Foreign air speed delivery is included in all *Clinics* subscription prices. All prices are subject to change without notice. **POSTMASTER:** Send address changes to *Oral and Maxillofacial Surgery Clinics of North America,* Elsevier Periodicals **Customer Service, 11830 Westline Industrial Drive, St. Louis, MO 63146. Tel: 1-800-654-2452 (U.S. and Canada); 314-447-8871 (outside U.S. and Canada). Fax: 314-447-8029. E-mail: journalscustomerservice-usa@elsevier.com (for print support); journalsonlinesupport-usa@elsevier.com (for online support).**

Reprints. For copies of 100 or more, of articles in this publication, please contact the Commercial Reprints Department, Elsevier Inc., 360 Park Avenue South, New York, NY 10010-1710. Tel.: 212-633-3874; Fax: 212-633-3820; Email: reprints@elsevier.com.

Oral and Maxillofacial Surgery Clinics of North America is covered in *MEDLINE/PubMed* (*Index Medicus*), *Science Citation Index Expanded* (*SciSearch®*), *Journal Citation Reports/Science Edition*, and *Current Contents®/Clinical Medicine*.

Contributors

CONSULTING EDITOR

RUI P. FERNANDES, MD, DMD, FACS, FRCS(Ed)
Clinical Professor and Chief, Division of Head and Neck Surgery, Program Director, Head and Neck Oncologic Surgery and Microvascular Reconstruction Fellowship, Departments of Oral and Maxillofacial Surgery, Neurosurgery, and Orthopaedic Surgery and Rehabilitation, University of Florida Health Science Center, University of Florida College of Medicine, Jacksonville, Florida

EDITOR

SRINIVAS M. SUSARLA, DMD, MD, MPH, FAAP, FACS
Associate Professor of Oral and Maxillofacial Surgery, University of Washington School of Dentistry, Associate Professor of Surgery (Plastic), University of Washington School of Medicine, Craniomaxillofacial Surgeon, Craniofacial Center, Seattle Children's Hospital, Seattle, Washington

AUTHORS

CRAIG B. BIRGFELD, MD, MD, FACS
Associate Professor, Department of Surgery, Division of Plastic Surgery, University of Washington, Seattle Children's Hospital, Seattle, Washington

MATTHEW BLESSING, MD
Associate Professor, Department of Pediatrics, Division of Craniofacial Medicine, University of Washington, Seattle Children's Hospital, Seattle, Washington

KEVIN CHEN, MD
Division of Plastic and Maxillofacial Surgery, Children's Hospital Los Angeles, Los Angeles, California

MARK A. EGBERT, DDS, FACS
Associate Professor of Oral and Maxillofacial Surgery, University of Washington School of Dentistry, Associate Professor of Surgery (Plastic), University of Washington School of Medicine, Chief, Division of Oral and Maxillofacial Surgery, Craniofacial Center, Seattle Children's Hospital, Seattle, Washington

RUSSELL E. ETTINGER, MD
Department of Surgery, Division of Plastic Surgery, University of Washington School of Medicine and Craniofacial Center, Seattle Children's Hospital, Seattle, Washington

G. KYLE FULTON, MD
Louisiana State University School of Medicine,
New Orleans, Louisiana

EMILY R. GALLAGHER, MD, MPH, FAAP
Associate Professor, Department of Pediatrics,
Division of Craniofacial Medicine, Craniofacial
Center, Seattle Children's Hospital, University
of Washington, Seattle, Washington; Louisiana
State University School of Medicine,
New Orleans, Louisiana

ALISA O. GIRARD, MBS
Department of Plastic and Reconstructive
Surgery, Craniofacial Research Fellow, Johns
Hopkins University, Baltimore, Maryland

JEFFREY A. HAMMOUDEH, MD, DDS
Division of Plastic and Maxillofacial Surgery,
Children's Hospital Los Angeles, Division of
Plastic and Reconstructive Surgery, Keck
School of Medicine of USC, Herman Ostrow
School of Dentistry, Division of Oral and
Maxillofacial Surgery, University of Southern
California, Los Angeles, California

JESSE T. HAN, DDS, MD
Resident, Department of Oral and Maxillofacial
Surgery, University of Washington School of
Dentistry, Seattle, Washington

GABRIEL M. HAYEK, DMD, MD
Division of Oral and Maxillofacial Surgery,
Department of Craniofacial Sciences,
University of Connecticut, Farmington,
Connecticut

TYLER J. HOLLEY, MD, DDS
Assistant Professor, Department of Oral and
Maxillofacial Surgery, The University of
Tennessee Medical Center, Knoxville,
Tennessee

RICHARD A. HOPPER, MD, MS, FACS
Marlys C. Larson Professor of Craniofacial
Surgery, University of Washington School of
Medicine, Chief, Division of Plastic and
Craniofacial Surgery and Surgical Director,
Craniofacial Center, Seattle Children's
Hospital, Seattle, Washington

DAVID F. JIMENEZ, MD, FACS
Director, Pediatric Neurosurgery, El Paso
Children's Hospital, El Paso, Texas

HITESH P. KAPADIA, DDS, PhD
Department of Surgery, Division of Plastic
Surgery, University of Washington School of
Medicine, Chief, Division of Craniofacial
Orthodontics, Craniofacial Center, Seattle
Children's Hospital, Seattle, Washington

KATELYN KONDRA, MD
Division of Plastic and Maxillofacial Surgery,
Children's Hospital Los Angeles, Los Angeles,
California

AMY LEE, MD, FAANS
Associate Professor of Neurosurgery,
University of Washington School of Medicine,
Chief, Division of Neurosurgery, Seattle
Children's Hospital Seattle, Washington

MICHAEL R. MARKIEWICZ, DDS, MPH, MD, FAAP, FRCD(c), FACS
Professor and Chair, Department of Oral and
Maxillofacial Surgery, William M. Feagans
Endowed Chair, Associate Dean for Hospital
Affairs, School of Dental Medicine, University
at Buffalo, Clinical Professor, Department of
Neurosurgery, Division of Pediatric Surgery,
Department of Surgery, Jacobs School of
Medicine and Biomedical Sciences, Co-
Director, Craniofacial Center of Western New
York, John Oishei Children's Hospital, Buffalo,
New York

BENJAMIN B. MASSENBURG, MD
Plastic Surgery Resident, University of
Washington School of Medicine, Seattle,
Washington

ERIC NAGENGAST, MD, MPH
Division of Plastic and Reconstructive Surgery,
Keck School of Medicine of USC, Los Angeles,
California

NATHAN J. RANALLI, MD, FAANS
Associate Professor of Neurosurgery and
Pediatrics, Associate Program Director of
Pediatric Craniofacial Surgery Fellowship,
Division of Pediatric Neurological Surgery,
University of Florida, Jacksonville,
Jacksonville, Florida

MATTHEW J. RECKER, MD
Resident in Training, Department of
Neurosurgery, Jacobs School of Medicine and
Biomedical Sciences, Buffalo, New York

RENÉE M. REYNOLDS, MD
Associate Professor and Program Director,
Department of Neurosurgery, Jacobs School
of Medicine and Biomedical Sciences, Buffalo,
New York

MELISSA ROY, MD
University of Washington, Seattle Children's
Hospital, Seattle, Washington

SAMEER SHAKIR, MD
Acting Instructor, University of Washington,
Seattle Children's Hospital, Seattle,
Washington

BARRY STEINBERG, MD, DDS, PhD, FACS
Professor and Director, Pediatric Craniofacial
Surgery Fellowship, Department of Oral and
Maxillofacial Surgery, University of Florida,
Gainesville, Gainesville, Florida

**SRINIVAS M. SUSARLA, DMD, MD, MPH,
FAAP, FACS**
Associate Professor of Oral and Maxillofacial
Surgery, University of Washington School of
Dentistry, Associate Professor of Surgery
(Plastic), University of Washington School of
Medicine, Craniomaxillofacial Surgeon,
Craniofacial Center, Seattle Children's
Hospital, Seattle, Washington

PHILIP D. TOLLEY, MD
Plastic Surgery Resident, University of
Washington School of Medicine, Seattle,
Washington

MARK M. URATA, MD, DDS
Division of Plastic and Maxillofacial Surgery,
Children's Hospital Los Angeles, Division
of Plastic and Reconstructive Surgery,
Keck School of Medicine of USC, Herman
Ostrow School of Dentistry, Division of Oral
and Maxillofacial Surgery, University
of Southern California, Los Angeles,
California

ROBIN YANG, MD, DDS
Assistant Professor, Department of Plastic and
Reconstructive Surgery, Director of Pediatric
Craniofacial Surgery, Chief of Oral and
Maxillofacial Surgery, Johns Hopkins Hospital,
Baltimore, Maryland

DAVID M. YATES, DMD, MD, FACS
Medical Director Cleft and Craniofacial
Surgery, Program Director, EPCH Cleft and
Craniofacial Fellowship, El Paso Children's
Hospital, Partner, High Desert Oral and Facial
Surgery, El Paso, Texas

Contents

The history of craniofacial surgery is one of many fundamental advances by monumental figures. Although craniosynostosis has been known to exist for multiple centuries, modern management has evolved over roughly the last century. An overview of early history, early scientific exploration, the advancement of surgical treatment of craniofacial deformities and the current state of craniosynostosis management is discussed. To fully appreciate the evolution of craniosynostosis surgery, one must understand the gradual advancements that have brought the specialty to this modern era.

Craniosynostosis, the premature fusion of the infant cranial skulls, can be recognized by characteristic head shape differences that worsen with head growth. Craniosynostosis can be syndromic or nonsyndromic and can involve one suture or multiple sutures. Timely cranial vault surgery is recommended to expand and reshape the skull, with a goal of preventing increased intracranial pressure and providing sufficient space for brain growth. Several gene variants and environmental exposures are known to increase the risk of single suture craniosynostosis (SSC), including in utero constraint, exposure to specific toxins and medications, and medical conditions such as thyroid dysregulation and metabolic bone disorders.

Infants and children with craniosynostosis require multidisciplinary care, and this is best accomplished when care is provided on a craniofacial team. Most patients with craniosynostosis will have non-syndromic presentations; however, longitudinal care remains critical to ensure appropriate growth and development throughout childhood. In patients with syndromic craniosynostoses, coordinated longitudinal care becomes even more paramount because of the high level of complexity across many different specialties or disciplines. Care delivery that includes perspective and expertise from multiple disciplines is important to help patients reach their full potential and optimal outcomes.

Fronto-orbital advancement remains a powerful technique for the correction of anterior cranial vault differences related to metopic (trigonocephaly) or unilateral coronal (anterior plagiocephaly) craniosynostoses. Traditional fronto-orbital advancement requires access to the forehead and superior 2/3 of the orbit via a coronal incision. The frontal bone and orbital segment (bandeau) are then separated from the skull and reshaped.

In patients with metopic craniosynostosis, the bandeau and frontal bone will need to be advanced and widened. In patients with unilateral coronal craniosynostosis, the bandeau will need to be "untwisted" to address the supraorbital retrusion on the affected side, the affected orbit will need to be shortened and widened, and the frontal bone flap will need to be proportionately advanced on the affected side. Overcorrection of the affected dimension should be undertaken to account for growth and relapse.

Early endoscopic-assisted correction of unicoronal and metopic synostosis is an excellent, safe, cost-effective, and highly effective option for affected patients. Although open calvarial remodeling has a place in the armamentarium of the craniofacial team, the skull base changes seen in endoscopic-assisted techniques are unparalleled. The procedures are associated with low morbidity and no mortality. There is minimal blood loss, decreased operating time, significantly reduced blood transfusion rates, decreased hospitalization length, decreased cost, and less pain and swelling. Early diagnosis and referral for surgical evaluation are critical to obtaining these results.

The prevalence of sagittal and lambdoid suture craniosynostosis differs considerably, as they are notably the most and least prevalent sutures involved in isolated suture craniosynostosis, respectively. The goals of reconstructing the cranial vault in both entities is the same: to release the fused suture, expand cranial volume, restore normal head shape and morphology, and allow for normal growth of the cranial vault. With regards to sagittal suture synostosis, opinions vary on whether reconstruction should focus on either the anterior or poster cranial vault. In contrast, the poster cranial vault is always targeted in lambdoid suture craniosynostosis.

The resurgence of strip craniectomies began in the mid-1990s with advances in surgical technique and anesthesia coupled with the critical observation that earlier interventions benefitted from an easily molded skull. Jimenez and Barone's pioneering introduction of endoscopic approaches to strip craniectomies coupled with postoperative helmeting in newborns and young infants and Claes Lauritzen's introduction of spring-mediated cranioplasty began the era of minimally invasive approaches in the surgical correction of craniosynostosis. This article provides technical descriptions of these treatment modalities, a comparative literature review, and our institutional algorithms for the correction of sagittal craniosynostosis and unilambdoid craniosynostosis.

Although most reported cases of minor suture involvement include multiple sutures, isolated suture involvement has been reported. Morphologic differences such as scaphocephaly and anterior plagiocephaly have been reported. Management should involve proper identification and multidisciplinary treatment. Surgical treatment should involve the expansion of the cranial vault as well as the correction of the deformity.

Syndromic craniosynostosis (CS) represents a relatively uncommon disease process that poses significant reconstructive challenges for the craniofacial surgeon. Although there is considerable overlap in clinical features associated with various forms of syndromic CS, key extracranial features and close examination of the extremities help to distinguish the subtypes. While Virchow's law can easily guide the diagnosis of single suture, nonsyndromic CS, syndromic CS traditionally results in atypical presentations inherent to multiple suture fusion. Coronal ring involvement in isolation or associated with additional suture fusion is the most common pattern in syndromic CS often resulting in turribrachycephaly.

Frontofacial surgery, encompassing the monobloc with or without facial bipartition and the box osteotomy, can treat the frontal bone and midface simultaneously, providing comprehensive improvement in facial balance. Complex pediatric patients with genetic syndromes and craniosynostosis are most optimized by an interdisciplinary team of surgeons, pediatricians, geneticists, speech pathologists, audiologists, dietitians, pediatric dentists, orthodontists, and psychosocial support staff to manage the myriad of challenges and complications throughout early childhood and beyond. Despite early treatment of the anterior and posterior cranial vault, these patients frequently have resultant frontal and/or midface hypoplasia and orbital abnormalities that are best managed with simultaneous surgical treatment.

Patients with syndromic craniosynostosis can present with midface hypoplasia, abnormal facial ratios, and obstructive sleep apnea. These symptoms can all be improved with midface advancement, but it is essential to evaluate the specific morphologic characteristics of each patient's bony deficiencies before offering subcranial advancement. Midface hypoplasia in Crouzon syndrome is evenly distributed between the central and lateral midface and reliably corrected with Le Fort III distraction. In contrast, the midface hypoplasia in Apert/Pfeiffer syndromes occurs in both an axial and a sagittal plane, with significantly more nasomaxillary hypoplasia compared with the orbitozygomatic deficiency.

Patients with syndromic and nonsyndromic synostosis may have end-stage skeletal discrepancies involving the lower midface and mandible, with associated malocclusion. While orthognathic surgical procedures in this population can be reliably executed, the surgeon must be aware of the unique morphologic characteristics that accompany the primary diagnoses as well as the technical challenges associated with performing Le Fort I osteotomies in patients who have undergone prior subcranial midface distraction.

ORAL AND MAXILLOFACIAL SURGERY CLINICS OF NORTH AMERICA

SERIES OF RELATED INTEREST

Atlas of the Oral and Maxillofacial Surgery Clinics
www.oralmaxsurgeryatlas.theclinics.com

Dental Clinics
www.dental.theclinics.com

THE CLINICS ARE NOW AVAILABLE ONLINE!
Access your subscription at:
www.theclinics.com

Preface
Craniosynostosis: Current Perspectives

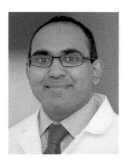

Srinivas M. Susarla, DMD, MD, MPH, FAAP, FACS
Editor

This issue of the *Oral and Maxillofacial Surgery Clinics of North America* focuses on the contemporary management of craniosynostosis. Craniosynostosis remains a diagnosis not infrequently encountered by the practicing oral and maxillofacial surgeon, whether in the context of providing craniofacial surgical care in infancy, adjunctive procedures during dentofacial development, or orthognathic surgery at skeletal maturity. In this regard, oral and maxillofacial surgeons play a key role in the longitudinal management of patients with craniosynostosis.

We are fortunate in this issue to have a diverse set of authors representing the multitude of specialists involved in care for this patient population. There is no doubt that patients with craniosynostosis are best served by multidisciplinary teams who work collaboratively to develop short- and long-term clinical care plans, effectively enact those plans, and continually assess their outcomes as a core component of process improvement. The contributions in this issue have been meticulously crafted to demonstrate that message. I remain indebted to our expert authors, who have taken time away from their professional and personal commitments to provide outstanding contributions that provide a primer for care from diagnosis in infancy to surgical management at skeletal maturity, illustrate historical perspectives on management, and discuss areas of active investigation. It is my hope that this issue will serve as a high-yield reference for the surgical practitioner caring for this patient population, regardless of the specific clinical context.

In addition to our contributors, there are a number of individuals who have helped this issue come to fruition. I would first like to thank Dr Rui Fernandes, who has been an outstanding friend and mentor, for helping me select this topic and develop the format for this issue. John Vassallo's robust experience with the *Oral and Maxillofacial Surgery Clinics of North America* and practical guidance helped facilitate an efficient process for the contributors. Jessica Cañaberal has been my closest professional partner with the day-to-day workflows that have ensured a high-quality product in a seamless manner.

Finally, I would like to thank my wife, Dr Harlyn Susarla, for her steadfast support as I committed time to this project, which took me away from her and our two lovely daughters. Her unwavering love, support, and advice have made all the difference in my career.

Srinivas M. Susarla, DMD, MD, MPH, FAAP, FACS
Seattle Children's Hospital
Craniofacial Center
4800 Sand Point Way NE
Seattle, WA 98105, USA

E-mail address:
srinivas.susarla@seattlechildrens.org

Oral Maxillofacial Surg Clin N Am 34 (2022) xi
https://doi.org/10.1016/j.coms.2022.06.005
1042-3699/22/© 2022 Published by Elsevier Inc.

oralmaxsurgery.theclinics.com

Historical Perspectives on the Management of Craniosynostosis

Tyler J. Holley, MD, DDS[a], Nathan J. Ranalli, MD[b],
Barry Steinberg, MD, DDS, PhD[c],*

KEYWORDS

• Craniosynostosis • Craniofacial surgery • Reconstruction • History

KEY POINTS

- An understanding of the history of surgical management of craniosynostosis is vital for the comprehension of the current state of craniosynostosis management.
- The evolution of craniosynostosis management has evolved from primitive approaches in the early historical period to advancement of surgical treatment in the current state of craniosynostosis.
- The management of patients with craniosynostosis continues to be an evolving discipline.

The history of craniofacial surgery is one of many fundamental advances by monumental figures. Although craniosynostosis has been known to exist for multiple centuries, modern management has evolved over roughly the last century. The confluence of multiple surgical specialties takes place in the treatment of craniosynostosis. As a result of their conjoint evolution the pioneers in the subspecialty of craniofacial surgery have established a firm surgical footing. To fully appreciate the evolution of craniosynostosis surgery, one must understand the gradual advancements that have brought the specialty to this modern era.

EARLY HISTORY PERIOD

It is the goal of the modern multidisciplinary craniofacial surgical team to restore anatomic form and function to the craniofacial unit. Historically, however, skull and facial deformity was the aim of different forms of cranial surgery, and craniofacial deformation techniques took place in many parts of the ancient world.[1–4] Deformation techniques included applying pads, stones, or board to the child's head to form it to a desired shape (**Fig. 1**). In addition, bandaging or binding were also used to deform the skull. Little evidence for the explanation of why deformation of the cranial skeleton was performed is known. However, several theories have been advanced[5]: (1) local cultural views of beauty, (2) tribal identity, (3) provision of a more ferocious and terrifying image of a warrior, (4) belief among the Incas that flattened foreheads made children more obedient, and (5) permission that was granted only to noble Peruvian families to shape their children's heads in the same fashion as their leaders.

Trephination was also performed in many parts of the world, with the earliest evidence showing that the procedure was being performed in the Neolithic Age.[6,7] It is thought that trephining was performed in attempts to treat epilepsy, insanity, unrelenting headaches, and other diseases. The goal of this surgery was perhaps to allow the "evil spirits" to escape via the trephine.[5] Examples of surgically treated skulls can be found in Germany, France, Peru, the Americas, and Ancient Egypt.[6,7]

[a] Department of Oral and Maxillofacial Surgery, University of Tennessee Medical Center, 1930 Alcoa Highway, Suite 335, Knoxville, TN 37920, USA; [b] Division of Pediatric Neurological Surgery, University of Florida, Jacksonville, 836 Prudential Drive, Pavilion Building Suite 1205, Jacksonville, FL 32207, USA; [c] Department of Oral and Maxillofacial Surgery, University of Florida, Jacksonville, 653-1 West 8th Street, Jacksonville, FL 32209, USA
* Corresponding author.
E-mail address: barry.steinberg@jax.ufl.edu

Oral Maxillofacial Surg Clin N Am 34 (2022) 333–340
https://doi.org/10.1016/j.coms.2022.01.004
1042-3699/22/© 2022 Elsevier Inc. All rights reserved.

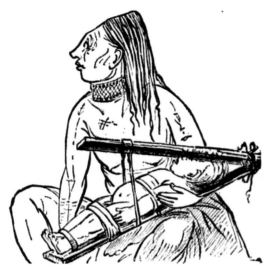

Fig. 1. Example of Chinook child with cradle board applied to form the head into the desired shape. (*From* Mason OT. Cradles of the American aborigines. Annual Report Smithsonian Institute Washington, DC. US Government Printing Office. 1889.)

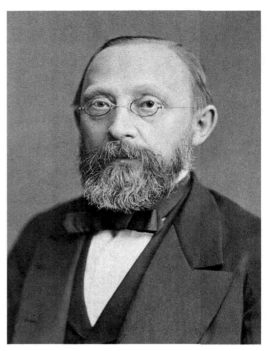

Fig. 2. Rudolf Ludwig Carl Virchow. (*From* The National Library of Medicine)

EARLY SCIENTIFIC EXPLORATION

Hippocrates was born around 460 BC on the island of Cos and died at Larissa in Thessaly about 377 BC. One of his greatest contributions to medicine was the idea that illness was a natural process and that the role of the physician was to aid the body in natural recovery. He provided one of the earliest descriptions of deformation of various cranial sutures and resultant head shapes in his *Collected Works*.[8] This book was translated to English by Francis Adams who named the collection *Genuine Works*.[9] An example of the description is as follows:

"Men's heads are by no means all like to one another, nor are the sutures of the head of all men constructed in the same form. Thus, whoever has a prominence in the anterior part of the head, in him the sutures of the head take the form of the Greek letter Tau T: for the head has the shorter line running transverse before the prominence, while the other line runs through the middle of the head, all the way to the neck... But whoever has a prominence of the head both before and behind, in him the sutures resemble the Greek letter eta H; [in Greek the letter H is rotated 90 degrees] for the long lines of the letter run transverse before each prominence while the short one runs through the middle and terminates in the long lines. But whoever has no prominence on either part he has the sutures of the head resembling the Greek letter X; for the one line comes transverse to the temple while the other passes along the middle of the head."

The German physician Samuel Thomas von Sömmerring (1755–1830) proposed that cranial sutures were present to allow for brain growth.[10] He made the astute hypothesis that if a suture closed prematurely abnormal head shape and cranial growth would result. In his writings he described the primary defect and sought to determine the global cranial impact. He was also one of the first to describe a case of lambdoid craniosynostosis. Soon after, the German anatomist Adolph Wilhem Otto (1786–1845), a specialist in the field of teratology, was credited for first coining the term *craniosynostosis* in 1830.[11] He proposed that one of the consequences of premature suture fusion was compensatory cranial expansion along another vector.[12] Basing his observations on both humans and animals, he provided the first explanation for global congenital cranial anomalies.

Rudolf Ludwig Carl Virchow (1821–1902) was a German physician who is known as "the father of modern pathology" and was primarily interested in the study of cretinism (**Fig. 2**). In 1851 he published his landmark paper in which he described the fundamental aberrant growth patterns in craniosynostosis (Virchow law).[13] Virchow law stated that the observed deformities occurred as a result of cessation of growth across a prematurely fused suture with compensatory growth along nonfused sutures in a direction parallel to the affected suture. This phenomenon would lead to obstruction of normal brain growth[14]; this is accepted as being the first accurate global principle applicable to all patterns of premature suture fusion. Virchow's authority as a pathologist led to widespread acceptance of his descriptions and mechanistic theories of premature suture fusion causing skull abnormalities. Virchow's contribution to the treatment of craniosynostosis cannot be overstated as the first surgical interventions and further iterations were based directly on his observations and principles of pathophysiology. By the early 1900s, the theory that craniosynostosis was a component of complex syndromic deformities gained traction. Apert (in 1906)[15] and Crouzon (in 1912)[16] described and named 2 of the most well-known syndromic deformities.

At the age of 21, René Le Fort (1869–1951) became the youngest in Frenchman to receive a Doctor of Medicine[17] (**Fig. 3**). After completing his residency be began his career as a military surgeon. In 3 consecutive issues of *Revue de Chirurgie* in 1901, he published on fractures of the facial skeleton.[18] Using cadavers, he applied a variety of forces to different regions of the facial skeleton. These forces vary from a heel of his boot to a wooden club, and in some experiments a cadaveric head was thrown at the edge of a wooden table. Once the force was applied, he then removed the soft tissue by boiling the heads and proceeded to meticulously examine and record the fracture patterns that were present. In the final of 3 papers, Le Fort summarized his work by detailing the "great lines of weakness," which corresponded to today's nomenclature of Le Fort I, II, and III fracture patterns.[18]

During World War I Le Fort, while serving as a military surgeon, became interested in thoracic surgery and published a book on penetrating thoracic injuries.[19] After the war he returned home and became interested in orthopedic surgery and was later elected President of the French Society of Orthopedics. Le Fort's work has served as a hallmark for future explorations in craniomaxillofacial surgery; this was not only in traumatology, but also for facial osteotomies to correct craniofacial abnormalities. It has been stated that "if Tessier is the father of craniofacial surgery, it should be acknowledged that Le Fort was the grandfather."[19]

ADVANCEMENT OF SURGICAL TREATMENT OF CRANIOFACIAL DEFORMITIES

Toward the end of the nineteenth century several reports of surgical treatments of craniosynostosis were described. Notably, LC Lane (1830–1902) of San Francisco reported that a mother of a child with microcephaly asked him "Can you not unlock my poor child's brain and let it grow"?[20] Lane intervened and performed a series of strip craniectomies, including removal of a stenosed sagittal suture and paired lateral strips of bone bilaterally. However, the child died within 48 hours, reportedly of anesthetic complications. Despite this, the described technique was quickly adopted and used for treatment of craniosynostosis (**Fig. 4**). Of great historic importance, the differentiation of microcephaly from craniosynostosis was poorly understood at the time, and the resulting outcomes of these procedure were often questioned. Additionally, these procedures were routinely performed after neurologic deficits had already developed and resolution of symptoms was often not seen. In response to their prior outcomes, Abraham Jacobi (1830–1919), a revered New York pediatrician, reviewed a series of 33 children treated for craniosynostosis. He found alarming results of surgery (15 of 33 children died as a result of the procedures). He denounced the

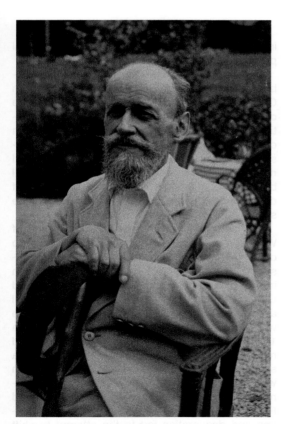

Fig. 3. René Le Fort. (René Léon Le Fort. Photograph, 1943 (?). Wellcome Collection..)

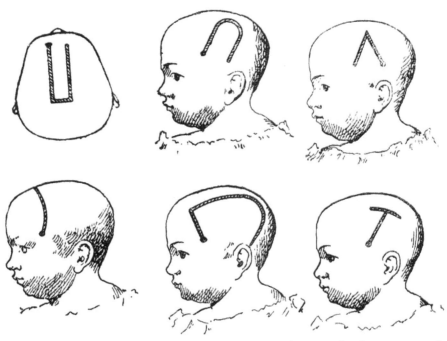

Fig. 4. Example of strip craniectomy technique used in late nineteenth century for the treatment of craniosynostosis. (*From* Padula F. Chirurgia Cranica. Le operazioni che si praticano sulle ossa del cranio. Rome, Dante Laighiere, 1895.)

craniectomies as harmful, excessively used, and of doubtful benefit in treatment of children.[21] He went on to say in his address entitled *Non nocere* (do no harm), "The relative impunity of operative interference accomplished by modern asepsis and antisepsis has developed an undue tendency to, and rashness in, handling the knife. The hands take too frequently the place of brains... Is it sufficient glory to don a white apron and swing a carbonized knife, and is therein a sufficient indication to let daylight into a deformed cranium and on top of the hopelessly defective brain, and to proclaim a success because the victim consented not to die of the assault? Such rash feats of indiscriminate surgery... are stains on your hands and sins on your soul. No ocean of soap and water will clean those hands, no power of corrosive sublimate will disinfect the souls."[21]

Despite this scathing rebuke, craniofacial surgeons continued to develop concepts for the management of craniofacial disorders. Additionally, anesthetic techniques improved and better control of blood loss was achieved.[5] In 1927 Faber and Towne,[22] now presumably with the capability to accurately differentiate microcephaly from craniosynostosis, argued for prevention of blindness and developmental delay by prophylactic craniotomies in children with elevated intracranial pressures. Their work led to an improved outcome with increased efficacy and safety of craniofacial procedures.

In the 1940s strip craniectomies were popularized again by the group of surgeons at Boston Children's Hospital. This group's focus was one of addressing the limitations of surgical intervention for children who experienced reossification of the craniectomy site and for children who presented late in the disease course.[23,24] Additional modifications included removing additional cranial bone, experimenting with different directions of craniotomies, adding interpositional polyurethane sheets, and usage of Zenker solution.[25,26]

The devastating craniomaxillofacial injuries of World War II offered another opportunity to develop techniques for craniomaxillofacial reconstruction. Through his extensive experience with injuries of the face as a result of combat, Sir Harold Gillies of Britain (1882–1960) was well versed in all aspects of facial reconstruction (**Fig. 5**). After the war, Gillies and Harrison[27] described a case of a 14-year-old girl with turricephaly, exorbitism, and midfacial hypoplasia (**Fig. 6**). The potential for a successful outcome was based on a discussion with a neurosurgeon who established that the cerebrospinal fluid pressure was normal. The "Grand Remedy" was begun, and a "blending of inspiration and desperation led to the attempt to shift her whole bony face and palate forward en

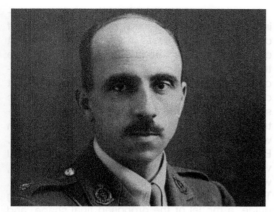

Fig. 5. Sir Harold Gillies. (*Reproduced* with permission. Copyright Queen Mary's Hospital Archive.)

bloc."[28] After multiple osteotomies at the Le Fort III level were performed through facial incisions, the face was then advanced without use of interpositional grafts. Of note, the orbital cuts were forward on the orbital rim and the maxilla was divided through the pterygomaxillary fissure and the hard palate. The result was a correction of the exorbitism, midfacial hypoplasia, and overall facial appearance (**Fig. 7**). The "Grand Remedy" was the first description of a Le Fort III osteotomy

and a seminal case in the history of craniofacial surgery.

Paul Tessier (1917–2008) was a French surgeon who received training in maxillofacial, ophthalmic, and plastic surgery. While at Hospital Foch, he was presented a patient with Crouzon syndrome, exhibiting exorbitism and maxillary retrusion. He was aware of the 1950 case report by Gillies and set out to study the problems of moving the face en bloc, in an attempt to correct the entirety of facial abnormalities in one procedure. He began cadaver dissections in Nantes at night, traveling back and forth while working in Paris. After his preparation, he agreed to operate a patient with the deformities described earlier. When he performed his first Le Fort III-type procedure, Tessier's surgical plan differed from that of Gillies in that he performed a pterygomaxillary disjunction, rather than a transpalatal osteotomy. The orbital osteotomies were made posterior to the lacrimal groove and autogenous bone graft was interposed into the surgically created skeletal gaps.[19,29] He noted improved position of the globe and improved midfacial hypoplasia.

Soon after beginning his Le Fort III-type procedures, Tessier was presented with several patients with severe orbital hypertelorism. He discussed the possibility of a transcranial approach with

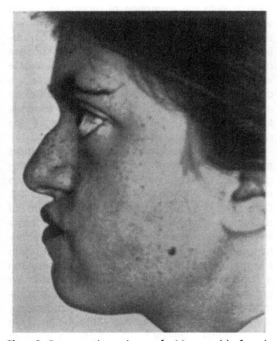

Fig. 6. Preoperative view of 14-year-old female demonstrating turricephaly, exorbitism, and midfacial hypoplasia. (*From* Gillies H, Harrison SH. Operative correction by osteotomy of recessed malar maxillary compound in a case of oxycephaly. Br J Plast Surg. 1950 Jul;3(2):123-7.)

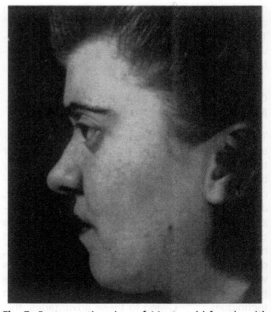

Fig. 7. Postoperative view of 14-year-old female with correction of exorbitism, midfacial hypoplasia, and overall facial appearance. (*From* Gillies H, Harrison SH. Operative correction by osteotomy of recessed malar maxillary compound in a case of oxycephaly. Br J Plast Surg. 1950 Jul;3(2):123-7.)

Gerard Guiot, a neurosurgical colleague at Hospital Foch.[19] Following their discussions and anatomic dissections, they embarked on the first transcranial approach for correction of hypertelorism. They approached through the anterior cranial base. The orbits were mobilized, which was followed by resection of the excess interorbital bone and correction of the hypertelorism[30]; this marked a big step forward for craniofacial surgery. In addition, another conceptual advance was described as the "useful orbit." The region is a centimeter in front of the optic foramen and behind the lacrimal groove.

Tessier's[31] perpetual drive to improve upon the techniques of craniofacial surgery led him to develop the concept of advancing the "orbitofrontal bandeau" and culminated in describing the facial bipartition procedure. The acronym SMAS (superficial musculoaponeurotic system) was introduced by Tessier in 1974. He also published the widely accepted classification of facial clefting syndromes.[32] It is not possible to completely document Tessier's contributions to the specialty of craniofacial surgery in this review; fortunately this has already been done.[33]

Adding to the work of Gillies and Tessier, Fernando Ortiz-Monasterio (1923–2012) further refined the treatment of midface hypoplasia associated with disorders such as Crouzon and Apert syndromes. He pioneered the monobloc advancement in which the orbits and midface advance in one piece combined with frontal repositioning.[34] The advantage of this technique is its ability to provide correction of the orbital asymmetry and midface retrusion during a single procedure.

CURRENT STATE OF CRANIOSYNOSTOSIS MANAGEMENT

The management of patients with craniosynostosis continues to be an evolving discipline. Over the last 2 decades endoscopy has increasingly been used in craniosynostosis surgery. In recognizing the limitations of open cranial vault surgery, Jimenez and Barone[35] introduced endoscopic-assisted strip craniectomies with postoperative cranial orthotic molding in 1998. Their method has demonstrated decreased operating time, decrease blood loss, and smaller surgical scars while providing end treatment results comparable to traditional open cranial vault reconstruction techniques.[36–41] Owing to these advantages, this less invasive approach has been adopted for specific cases by many craniofacial teams. However, this method of treatment heavily relies on patient/parent compliance and competence/presence of a local cranial orthotist.

The open techniques of cranial vault remodeling that were developed by the pioneers of craniofacial surgery still apply to the treatment of craniosynostosis today. Surgeons now have the capability of 3-dimensional analysis and preoperative virtual surgical planning in the treatment of craniosynostosis. Computed tomographic scans are uploaded to a medical modeling system in advance of the treatment planning session with outlines of the proposed osteotomies. Biomedical engineers then complete the virtual vault reshaping as directed by the surgeons, who subsequently approve the final product. Three models are often requested, a cutting guide, a model of the proposed final shape, and a model of the inner surface of the final shape. Three-dimensional analysis and virtual surgical planning have been theorized to improve the accuracy, operative efficiency, and reproducibility in craniofacial surgery.[42–44]

The first cases of distraction osteogenesis of the craniomaxillofacial skeleton were performed in 1926 and 1927 by the German craniofacial surgeons Wolfgang Rosenthal and Martin Wassmund, respectively.[45] Distraction osteogenesis of the mandible was described by Rosenthal and in the maxilla by Wassmund. Their techniques were further described in Wassmund's textbook in 1936.[46] With the exception of reports of palatal expansion (distraction) in the orthodontic literature, the technique seemed forgotten until the 1973 publication by Chifford Snyder[47] who reported success of distraction of a canine mandible. The technique was then later reintroduced by the clinical reports of Karp and colleagues[48] in 1990 and McCarthy and colleagues[49] in 1992, demonstrating osseous formation with distraction osteogenesis of the mandible.

Since the reintroduction in the 1990s, multiple adaptations have been made in distraction osteogenesis of the craniomaxillofacial skeleton for the treatment of craniosynostosis and its sequelae. Chin and Toth[50] described the first report of distraction osteogenesis of a Le Fort III osteotomy in 1996. The midface has been shown to be effectively advanced at the Le Fort III level using both internal and external distractors. Compared with a conventional osteotomy, distraction allows for greater overall advancement, the gradual accommodation of periorbital and perioral soft tissues, and the ability to control the vector when using an external device.[51] Similarly, monobloc advancement by distraction osteogenesis has been shown to have a lower complication rate, the ability to advance the midface further, and less relapse when compared with a conventional monobloc advancement procedure.[52,53]

In 2009 White and colleagues[54] published their initial experience with distraction osteogenesis of the posterior cranial vault. The technique has been shown to provide increased intracranial volume expansion when compared with fronto-orbital advancement and provides gradual expansion of the soft tissue envelope, potentially decreasing relapse.[55,56] Improved anterior and posterior cranial morphology as a result of posterior cranial vault distraction has also been reported.[56] Many centers have adopted this technique using posterior cranial vault distraction as the initial cranial remodeling procedure in syndromic craniosynostosis. This is not without controversy as posterior cranial vault distraction may necessitate intervention on unaffected cranial sutures and requires a secondary procedure for distractor removal.[57]

In the study of the history of craniosynostosis management one will note that the examples of surgical advancements have come through passion, devotion, and tireless efforts of the pioneers that came before us. As the science and art of craniosynostosis management progresses further, advancement will undoubtedly follow suit.

DISCLOSURE

None of the authors have any commercial or financial conflicts of interest or funding sources.

REFERENCES

1. Flower WH. Fashion in deformity, as illustrated in the customs of barbarous and civilized races. In: Humboldt library of popular science literaturevol. 2. New York: Fitzgerald; 1882. p. 1–49.
2. Gerszten PC. An investigation into the practice of cranial deformation among the pre-Columbian peoples of Northern Chile. Int J Osteoarcheol 1993;3:87.
3. Gerszten PC, Gerszten E. Intentional cranial deformation: A disappearing form of self-mutilation. Neurosurgery 1995;37:374.
4. Porter JH. Notes on the artificial deformation of children among savage and civilized peoples. Annual report of the Smithsonian Institute. Washington, Government Printing Office; 1889. p. 4.
5. Goodrich JT, Tutino M. An annotated history of craniofacial surgery and intentional cranial deformation. Neurosurg Clin N Am 2001;12(1):45–68, viii.
6. Davis JB. Thesaurus Craniorum. Catalogue of the skulls of various races of man. London: printed for subscribers; 1867.
7. Shapiro HL. A correction for artificial deformation of skulls. Anthropologic Pap Am Mus Nat Hist 1928; 30:1.
8. Hippocrates, Jones WHS. Hippocrates collected works. Cambridge Harvard University Press; 1968.
9. Hippocrates. The genuine works of hippocrates. Translated by Francis Adams. London: Sydenham Society; 1849.
10. Sömmerring ST. Vom baue des menschlichen Korpers. Leipzig (Germany): Voss; 1800.
11. Francone V. Adolph Wilhelm Otto. Available at: https://www.whonamedit.com/doctor.cfm/1303.html. Accessed July 1, 2021.
12. Otto AW. Lehrbuch der Pathologischen Anatomie des Menschen und der Thiere. Berlin (Germany): Rücker; 1830.
13. Virchow R. Uber den Cretinismus, namentlich in Franken, und uber pathologische Schadelformen. Verh Phys Med Gesell Wurzburg 1851;2:230–71.
14. Andersson H, Gomes SP. Craniosynostosis. Review of the literature and indications for surgery. Acta Paediatr Scand 1968;57:47–54.
15. Apert E. De l'acrocéphalosyndactalie. Bull Soc Méd Paris 1906;23:1310–30.
16. Crouzon O. Dysostose cranio-faciale hereditaire. Bull Mem Soc Med Hop Paris 1912;33:545–55.
17. Tessier P. Biographical sketch of Rene Le Fort. Plast Reconstr Surg 1972;50(6):606–7.
18. Le Fort R. Etude experimental sur les fractures de la machoire superieure. Rev Chir 1901;23208.
19. Waterhouse N. The history of craniofacial surgery. Facial Plast Surg 1993;9(2):143–50.
20. Lane LC. Pioneer craniectomy for relief of mental imbecility due to premature sutural closure and microcephalus. JAMA 1892;18:49–50.
21. Jacobi A. Non Nocere Med Rec 1894;45:609–18.
22. Faber HK, Towne EB. Early craniectomy as a preventive measure in oxycephaly and allied conditions: with special reference to the prevention of blindness. Am J Med Sci 1927;173:701–11.
23. Ingraham FD, Alexander E Jr, Matson DD. Clinical studies in craniosynostosis analysis of 50 cases and description of a method of surgical treatment. Surgery 1948;24:518–41.
24. Shillito J Jr, Matson DD. Craniosynostosis: a review of 519 surgical patients. Pediatrics 1968;41:829–53.
25. Jane JA, Edgerton MT, Futrell JW, et al. Immediate correction of sagittal synostosis. J Neurosurg 1978; 49:705–10.
26. Stein SC, Schut L. Management of scaphocephaly. Surg Neurol 1977;7:153–5.
27. Gillies H, Harrison SH. Operative correction by osteotomy of recessed malar maxillary compound in a case of oxycephaly. Br J Plast Surg 1951;3:123–7.
28. Gillies H, Millard DRC Jr. The principles and art of plastic surgery. Boston Little (MA): Brown & Company; 1957.
29. Tessier P. The definitive plastic surgical treatment of the severe facial deformities of craniofacial dysostosis. Crouzon's and Apert's diseases. Plast Reconstr Surg 1971;48(5):419–42.

30. Tessier P, Guiot G, Rougerie J, et al. Cranio-naso-orbito-facial osteotomies. Hypertelorism Ann Chir Plast 1967;12(2):103–18.

31. Tessier P. Facial bipartition: A concept more than a procedure. In: Marchac D, editor. Craniofacial surgery. Berlin (Germany): Springer-Verlag; 1987. p. 1.

32. Tessier P. Anatomical classification of facial, craniofacial and laterofacial clefts. J Maxillofac Surg 1976;4:69.

33. Ghali MG, Srinivasan VM, Jea A, et al. Craniosynostosis surgery: the legacy of Paul Tessier. Neurosurg Focus 2014;36(4):1–8.

34. Ortiz-Monasterio F, del Campo AF, Carrillo A. Advancement of the orbits and the midface in one piece, combined with frontal repositioning, for the correction of Crouzon's deformities. Plast Reconstr Surg 1978;61(4):507–16.

35. Jimenez DF, Barone CM. Endoscopic craniectomy for early surgical correction of sagittal craniosynostosis. J Neurosurg 1998;88:77–81.

36. Jimenez D, Barone C. Blood loss after endoscopic strip craniectomy for craniosynostosis. J Neurosurg Anesthesiol 2000;12(1):60.

37. Shah MN, Kane AA, Petersen JD, et al. Endoscopically assisted versus open repair of sagittal craniosynostosis: the St. Louis Children's Hospital experience. J Neurosurg Pediatr 2011;8:165–70.

38. Jimenez DF, Barone CM. Endoscopic techniques for craniosynostosis. Atlas Oral Maxillofac Surg Clin North Am 2010;18(2):93–107.

39. Thompson DR, Zurakowski D, Haberkern CM, et al. Endoscopic versus open repair for craniosynostosis in infants using propensity score matching to compare outcomes: a multicenter study from the Pediatric Craniofacial Collaborative Group. Anesth Analg 2018;126:968–75.

40. Jimenez DF, Barone CM. Endoscopic technique for sagittal synostosis. Childs Nerv Syst 2012;28(9):1333–9.

41. Jimenez DF, Barone CM, McGee ME, et al. Endoscopy-assisted wide-vertex craniectomy, barrel stave osteotomies, and postoperative helmet molding therapy in the management of sagittal suture craniosynostosis. J Neurosurg 2004;100(5 Suppl Pediatrics):407–17.

42. Seruya M, Borsuk DE, Khalifian S, et al. Computer-Aided Design and Manufacturing in Craniosynostosis Surgery. J Craniofac Surg 2013;24(4):1100–5.

43. Steinbacher DM. Three-dimensional analysis and surgical planning in craniomaxillofacial surgery. J Oral Maxillofac Surg 2015;73(12 Suppl):S40–56.

44. Adolphs N, Haberl EJ, Liu W, et al. Virtual planning for craniomaxillofacial surgery–7 years of experience. J Craniomaxillofac Surg 2014;42(5):e289–95.

45. Hönig JF, Grohmann UA, Merten HA. Facial Bone Distraction Osteogenesis for Correction of Malocclusion. Plast Reconstr Surg January 2002;109(1):41–4.

46. Wassmund M. Lehrbuch der praktischen Chirurgie des Mundes und der Kiefer. Leipzig (Germany): Verlag Von Hermann Meusser; 1935.

47. Snyder CC, Levine GA, Swasson HM, et al. Mandibular lengthening by gradual distraction. Plast Reconstr Surg 1973;51(5):506–8.

48. Karp NS, Thorne CH, McCarthy JC, et al. Bone lengthening in the craniofacial skeleton. Ann Plast Surg 1990;24:231.

49. McCarthy JG, Schreiber J, Karp N, et al. Lengthening the human mandible by gradual distraction. Plast Reconstr Surg 1992;89:1.

50. Chin M, Toth BA. Distraction osteogenesis in maxillofacial surgery using internal devices: review of five cases. J Oral Maxillofac Surg 1996;54(1):45–53.

51. Malagon HH, Romo GW, Quintero Mosqueda FR, et al. Multivectorial, external halo-assisted midface distraction in patients with severe hypoplasia. J Craniofac Surg 2008;19(6):1663–9.

52. Bradley JP, Gabbay JS, Taub PJ, et al. Monobloc advancement by distraction osteogenesis decreases morbidity and relapse. Plast Reconstr Surg 2006;118(7):1585–97.

53. Raposo-Amaral CE, Denadai R, Zanco GL, et al. Long-term follow-up on bone stability and complication rate after monobloc advancement in syndromic craniosynostosis. Plast Reconstr Surg 2020;145(4):1025–34.

54. White N, Evans M, Dover MS, et al. Posterior calvarial vault expansion using distraction osteogenesis. Childs Nerv Syst 2009;25(2):231–6.

55. Derderian CA, Wink JD, McGrath JL, et al. Volumetric changes in cranial vault expansion: comparison of fronto-orbital advancement and posterior cranial vault distraction osteogenesis. Plast Reconstr Surg 2015;135(6):1665–72.

56. Goldstein JA, Paliga JT, Wink JD, et al. A craniometric analysis of posterior cranial vault distraction osteogenesis. Plast Reconstr Surg 2013;131(6):1367–75.

57. Swanson JW, Samra F, Bauder A, et al. An Algorithm for managing syndromic craniosynostosis using posterior vault distraction osteogenesis. Plast Reconstr Surg 2016;137(5):829e–41e.

Epidemiology, Genetics, and Pathophysiology of Craniosynostosis

Matthew Blessing, MD, Emily R. Gallagher, MD, MPH*

KEYWORDS

• Craniosynostosis • Infant skull • Infant suture • Infant head shape

KEY POINTS

- Craniosynostosis can be differentiated from benign head shapes that may share some characteristics based on predictable physical examination findings, illustrated in this article.
- Potential in utero exposures to some medications, maternal medical conditions, and uterine constraints are associated with an increased risk of single suture craniosynostosis (SSC).
- Several gene variants are associated with single suture and multi-suture craniosynostosis (MSC), although genetic testing may be reserved for specific clinical scenarios whereby a variant is more likely to be identified.

INTRODUCTION

Craniosynostosis is the premature fusion of suture(s) of the skull. It typically occurs in utero (primary craniosynostosis) and can be recognized by abnormal head shape.[1] Secondary craniosynostosis, or postnatal fusion, is also possible and may be more difficult to recognize. The major sutures of a normal newborn skull (**Fig. 1**) are composed of fibrous connective tissue which responds in a complex, incompletely understood way to extrinsic and intrinsic factors. Factors extrinsic to the sutures include underlying brain growth, restriction of growth of the fetal head, and environmental factors.[2] Intrinsic factors include embryologic cell growth, migration, and differentiation, which are influenced by numerous genes, some of which are likely undiscovered.[2]

Craniosynostosis can involve one suture or multiple sutures and can be an isolated problem (nonsyndromic craniosynostosis) or associated with other medical problems or a known gene variant (syndromic craniosynostosis). Craniosynostosis typically presents in a predictable manner because the expansion of the skull occurs whereby sutures are open and is restricted whereby sutures are closed, thereby resulting in characteristic head shape differences. When a single suture is fused prematurely, perpendicular growth is restricted, and brain growth, therefore, must expand the skull whereby the sutures remain open. In addition to describing and illustrating the head shape differences and facial features associated with single suture craniosynostosis (SSC), we will also present cases of multi-suture craniosynostosis (MSC). Patients with MSC are more likely to have an underlying gene variant[2,3] and may also have an increased risk of upper airway obstruction, malocclusion, or associated anatomic and medical problems.

Timely identification of craniosynostosis is essential because of its potential consequences on a child's health and quality of life. The sutures, when patent, enable cranial deformation during birth, allow sufficient bony protection for the brain during periods of rapid growth, and control cellular signaling involved in calvarial growth.[4] Untreated craniosynostosis can cause increased intracranial pressure,[5,6] leading to such consequences as chronic headaches,[7] developmental delay, and vision loss. Treatment of craniosynostosis involves a surgery to remodel the cranial vault and restore sufficient room for brain growth, while also

Department of Pediatrics, Division of Craniofacial Medicine, University of Washington and Seattle Children's Hospital, 4800 Sand Point Way NE, M/S OB.9.520, PO Box 5371, Seattle, WA 98145-5005, USA
* Corresponding author.
E-mail address: emily.gallagher@seattlechildrens.org

Oral Maxillofacial Surg Clin N Am 34 (2022) 341–352
https://doi.org/10.1016/j.coms.2022.02.001
1042-3699/22/© 2022 Elsevier Inc. All rights reserved.

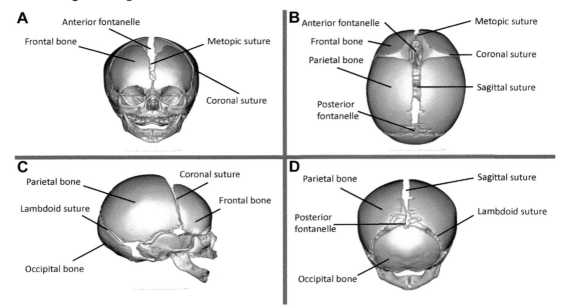

Fig. 1. Normal infant CT skull with (A) front, (B) top–down, (C) side, and (D) back view. Major sutures, bones, and fontanelles are labeled.

normalizing the shape of the skull. Depending on the suture involved, there are recommended time windows for intervention. If delayed beyond the recommended age, surgery will be associated with increased risks for the child. Even after surgery, there remains a slightly increased risk for lower scores on standardized evaluations of development, intelligence, and academic functioning, though these impacts are typically mild.[8–12] At this time, it is not possible to predict which patients with SSC will develop increased intracranial pressure and which will not. Additionally, directly measuring intracranial pressure is invasive. Monitoring for papilledema is helpful, but this is considered a late sign, when damage from the increased pressure has likely already occurred. It is essential to discuss these risks in detail with the child's caregiver(s) when counseling them about the risks and benefits of surgical intervention.

Here, we will discuss the epidemiology, genetics, and pathophysiology of craniosynostosis. The primary focus will be on SSC, but we will include considerations for MSC as well (sequential care for patients with MSC is discussed later in this volume). We will also discuss conditions that may resemble craniosynostosis but do not require surgery and explain how to differentiate. This review should equip the reader with the ability to counsel a family in detail and comfort them as they process this diagnosis and the recommended treatment.

Epidemiology and pathophysiology

Overall, SSC occurs in around 1 in 2500 births and comprises 80% of all cases of craniosynostosis.[1]

Compared with earlier studies of birth prevalence, the prevalence of craniosynostosis increased between 1999 and 2014 in the United States, Europe, and Australia. The most significant and consistent increase was seen with metopic craniosynostosis.[13,14] Although not fully understood, this may be due in part to improved awareness of the diagnosis by providers. However, the severity of presentation did not increase during this time, suggesting that other factors are involved. Sagittal craniosynostosis is the most common single suture to fuse and comprises around 50% of cases. After that, metopic is most common at 24% to 36%, followed by coronal at 11% and lambdoid at 0% to 2%.[15,16]

Several factors increase the risk of any SSC cases and are not clearly suture-specific. These include environmental exposures and mechanical forces. Some genetic variants are known to be associated with craniosynostosis, but these are often suture-specific.

Environmental exposures

Many environmental exposures associated with an increased risk of craniosynostosis apply to all sutures. Higher parental age increases the risk of craniosynostosis. This is usually related to maternal age, although advanced paternal age has also been implicated.[17] An association has also been seen with *in vitro* fertilization, although advanced maternal age is often confounding. Infants born to mothers who smoke have an increased risk of craniosynostosis, especially when mothers smoke 15 or more cigarettes per day and continue smoking after the first trimester.[18]

Several medication exposures have been found to increase the risk of SSC. Exposure to valproic acid (and likely other antiepileptics) during pregnancy has long been known to significantly increase the risk of SSC,[19–21] particularly metopic craniosynostosis. Exposure to nitrofurantoin has been less clearly associated with SSC but may still be of concern.[22,23] Exposure to sertraline during the first trimester of pregnancy is associated with an over 2-fold increased risk of craniosynostosis,[24] though this association is less clear for first trimester use of other selective serotonin reuptake inhibitors (SSRIs).[25]

Studies have evaluated whether nutrient intake during pregnancy may be associated with craniosynostosis, and the associations are not fully delineated but seem to vary by suture type. Folic acid intake has not been shown to be associated with fusion of any suture. The risk of sagittal craniosynostosis was lower among women with high first trimester intake of riboflavin and vitamins B_6, E, and C. High intake of vitamin C and methionine may reduce the risk of coronal craniosynostosis if taken early in pregnancy. High first trimester intakes of choline and vitamin B_{12}, however, may increase the risk of metopic craniosynostosis.[26] None of these findings from observational studies have led to changes in nutrition recommendations during pregnancy.

Infants of mothers with thyroid dysfunction are known to have an increased risk of craniosynostosis. The sagittal suture was most affected, followed by the coronal and then metopic. Using data from the National Birth Defects Prevention Study, researchers found that mothers of children with SSC were more than twice as likely to report thyroid disease (including Graves' disease and its treatment) compared with mothers of control infants.[27] Because thyroid disease is common among women of reproductive age and is not always diagnosed, later studies have investigated and found support for the association of risk factors for maternal thyroid dysfunction with craniosynostosis.[28] This is biologically plausible, as studies treating animal models with thyroid hormones stimulates osteogenesis and premature narrowing of the cranial sutures,[29] and clinically relevant as it is a treatable condition.

Metabolic bone disorders are associated with increased risk of secondary craniosynostosis. As mentioned above, secondary craniosynostosis develops postnatally and is often recognized at a later age because the head shape differences may not be as apparent. Rickets has long been known to be associated with craniosynostosis. Vitamin D is lacking in rickets, resulting in inadequate calcium and phosphorus in the bloodstream. Hypophosphatemic rickets, whereby phosphorus is depleted despite adequate intake of vitamin D and calcium, can be associated with inadequate absorption or increased losses from renal or gastrointestinal disorders, and there are also X-linked and autosomal dominant genetic etiologies.[30] Metabolic bone disorders are usually associated with sagittal craniosynostosis, but coronal, lambdoid, and pansynostosis have also been reported.[31] Other forms of metabolic disorders, such as hypophosphatasia, pseudohypoparathyroidism, osteopetrosis, and mucopolysaccharidosis disorders may also result in craniosynostosis.[31] Because of the later presentation of craniosynostosis of these disorders, the resultant head shape differences may not be apparent and surgical recommendations require more consideration. Patients should still be monitored for the development of increased intracranial pressure, and surgical recommendations should be discussed by a multidisciplinary team that includes expertise in skeletal disorders, in addition to craniofacial conditions.

Mechanical forces

Typical calvarial growth depends on the brain pushing outward on the calvarium causing skull growth and maintaining patency of the sutures.[32,33] Secondary craniosynostosis may result from abnormal brain growth. For example, an infant with hypoxic-ischemic encephalopathy resulting in limited brain growth, or an infant with hydrocephalus who has growth alterations following shunt placement with subsequent decompression may develop secondary craniosynostosis.[34] In addition, several studies have indicated that intrauterine constraint may cause primary craniosynostosis.[35] SSC is more common in cases of multiple births, bicornuate uterus, or intrauterine fibroids.

Genetics

In addition to the mechanical and environmental risks, genetic factors have also been implicated in SSC. While gene variants have been more clearly established in patients with syndromic craniosynostosis, several variants have also been identified in patients with SSC. One study of 391 participants with SSC found that 15% had potential causal variants in 29 genes.[36] Mutations associated with SSC are autosomal dominant around 8% of the time.[36,37] Genome-wide association studies have also identified genes involved in SSC.[38] Studying familial patterns of inheritance has shown differences by suture type, with highest incidence for first-degree relatives of probands with metopic craniosynostosis (6.4%), followed by sagittal (3.8%), lambdoid (3.9%), and coronal (0.7%).[39] Because of the large number of potential variants, genetic testing is typically not recommended for patients with SSC unless it is familial, the patient has a recognized syndrome, or the coronal suture is involved (as this is more clearly associated with a small number of variants).

Also supporting the role of genetics in SSC are differences in incidence based on gender or ethnicity. Sagittal and metopic craniosynostosis are more common in boys, while unilateral coronal craniosynostosis is more common in girls.[15,16] A study in the US of SSC and ethnicity found that Caucasians and African Americans were the predominant ethnic groups among all cases, with Caucasians more likely to have metopic craniosynostosis and African Americans more likely to present with unilateral coronal synostosis.[40] A European study comparing people with craniosynostosis of Caucasian or Asian descent found higher prevalence than expected in the Asian community.[41] Additional multinational studies are needed to validate these findings and understand the etiologies of the observed differences.

SINGLE SUTURE CRANIOSYNOSTOSIS
Sagittal craniosynostosis

The sagittal suture is the most common suture to fuse prematurely among all cases of SSC and comprises about 40% to 50% of all cases.[13] Males are more likely to be affected than females (75.2% and 24.8%, respectively[13]) for reasons that are not understood. The theories described above about constraint increasing the risk of craniosynostosis apply to sagittal craniosynostosis. Many studies have suggested that macrosomia (birth weight >4000 g) is predictive of an increased risk of sagittal synostosis.[14]

When the sagittal suture fuses prematurely the skull cannot expand its biparietal width, leading to elongation along the anterior–posterior direction with frontal bossing and occipital prominence (**Fig. 2**). The resulting long, narrow head shape is termed scaphocephaly. Normally the widest point of the skull is over the parietal bones. However, the head shape of sagittal craniosynostosis may have the widest part over the occipital or frontal bones, and the forehead and/or occiput may look more prominent. A palpable ridge is often present over the sagittal suture, and in some cases, the shape of the anterior fontanelle may feel more triangular than diamond shaped.

Breech positioning *in utero* can mimic scaphocephaly (**Fig. 3**A, B); however, this usually resolves after a few days in most cases. A ridge should not be present over the sagittal suture, although sometimes the parietal bones may be overlapping in the first few days, which may be confused for a ridge. To differentiate, the parietal bones should be easily ballotable across the suture, and this subtle movement confirms the patency of the suture. Bathrocephaly, a head shape with a prominence at the occipital bone causing a shelf-like protuberance, may also mimic scaphocephaly (**Fig. 3**C, D). This results from a patent mendosal suture, a fetal suture that runs across the occipital bone and usually fuses before birth. In some cases, the mendosal suture is persistently open, resulting in a place whereby the bone can protrude outward as the brain grows. This condition is benign, with no increased risk for increased

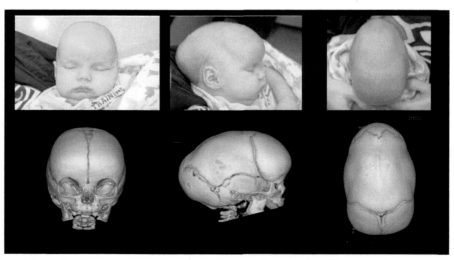

Fig. 2. Infant with sagittal craniosynostosis and resulting scaphocephaly, with narrowing along the skull and prominence of the occipital and frontal bones.

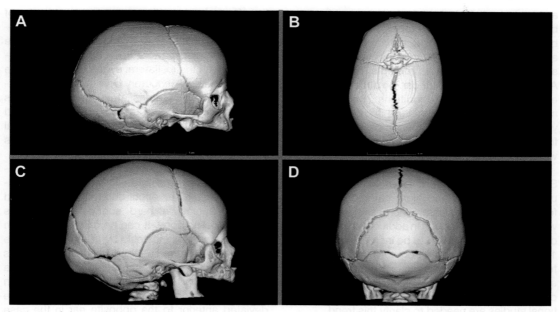

Fig. 3. Head shapes that may mimic scaphocephaly from sagittal craniosynostosis. (*A, B*) show a 3-month-old who had been breech *in utero*. Note the relative elongation of the skull with narrowing across the parietal bones. (*C, D*) show an infant with bathrocephaly, a shelf-like protrusion over the occipital bone with associated elongation because of a persistent mendosal suture, the fetal suture that bisects the occipital bone.

intracranial pressure. Indeed, it is quite the opposite of craniosynostosis.[42]

Metopic craniosynostosis

When the metopic suture fuses prematurely, the frontal bones cannot expand laterally, leading to a triangular shape to the forehead called trigonocephaly (**Fig. 4**). This shape of the forehead coincides with the distortion of the bony orbits as well, causing hypotelorism, raised or arched eyebrows, and lateral orbital hypoplasia.[43] Biparietal widening is also often present.

Metopic craniosynostosis may be confused with a metopic ridge, which is a benign variant. All the major sutures should be open until the second or third decade of life, with the exception of the metopic suture, which typically starts closing between 3 and 9 months of age.[44] When it is in the process of fusing, it often has a palpable ridge

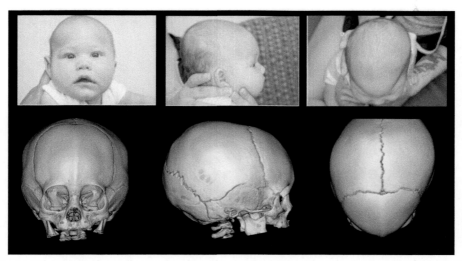

Fig. 4. Infant with metopic craniosynostosis showing trigonocephaly with hypotelorism, arched eyebrows, and deficient lateral orbits.

associated with it. A physiologic metopic ridge can be differentiated from metopic craniosynostosis because of the age of onset, the forehead contour, and facial features. While metopic craniosynostosis is treated surgically, metopic ridge is not. Although in some cases it can be difficult to differentiate between the conditions, patients with metopic craniosynostosis tend to present at a younger age, and the appearance of the lateral frontal bone and lateral orbit can help distinguish whether there is pathology.[43]

Many of the risk factors described above for all SSC apply to metopic craniosynostosis. In particular, multiple births and high maternal age were found to have significantly increased association with metopic synostosis.[14] In addition, while the incidence of SSC was found to be increasing between 1999 and 2014 from data from the Texas Birth Defects Registry, the increase was largest for metopic synostosis.[13] This may be related to associated increases in maternal characteristics, though additional studies are needed to clarify this trend.

Regarding genetic etiologies of metopic synostosis, routine genetic testing is not clearly indicated based on the large numbers of potential gene variants and low yield. However, in cases whereby an underlying syndrome is suspected, a chromosome microarray may be helpful. Several chromosomal abnormalities are associated with metopic craniosynostosis, including 9p23.3 deletion, 11q23.3 deletion, 1p36.3 duplication, 7p deletion, and others.[2]

Unicoronal craniosynostosis

When a single coronal suture fuses, it leads to forehead retrusion and distortion of the orbit on the affected side, with consequent asymmetry of the forehead that is best appreciated from a top–down view of the skull (**Fig. 5**). The eye on the affected side looks more open than the contralateral eye, with the ipsilateral eyebrow raised. There also may be compensatory bossing of the contralateral forehead. The ipsilateral glenoid fossa is displaced forward, and the chin can be deviated to the contralateral side. This seems as a facial twist toward the unaffected side, which worsens as the child grows.[45]

Deformational plagiocephaly, especially if present at birth, can present similarly to unicoronal craniosynostosis. It can occur due to the fetus's head pressing against a hard surface, such as its mother's pelvic bone. It can be differentiated from unicoronal craniosynostosis by the position of the ear ipsilateral to the flattened forehead, as well as the shape of the ipsilateral orbit. The ear on the affected side will be posterior to the other ear in the case of deformational changes, while it will be deviated anterior to the opposite ear in the case of unicoronal craniosynostosis. The ipsilateral orbit does not look larger in the case of deformational changes, as it does in unicoronal craniosynostosis.[45] Furthermore, the head shape and facial features of a child with unicoronal craniosynostosis will become more obvious with time, while deformational plagiocephaly typically improves with age in a child who is typically developing.

Unicoronal craniosynostosis is the third most common SSC, following sagittal and metopic. It occurs in approximately 1 out of every 10,000 live births.[45] It occurs more frequently in women than men, which sets it apart from sagittal and metopic craniosynostosis.[13] In terms of fetal constraint, one

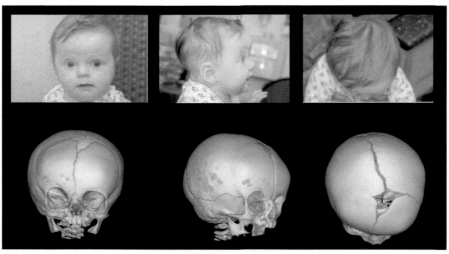

Fig. 5. Infant with right unicoronal craniosynostosis. Note the right anterior flattening with orbital retrusion and facial twist to the contralateral side.

study showed a nearly 2-fold increase of unicoronal craniosynostosis if the fetus had macrosomia.[35]

Unicoronal craniosynostosis is the SSC most likely to be caused by an identifiable underlying genetic difference, with studies showing that 10% to 30% of patients have a variant that can be detected.[3] Common gene variants associated with unicoronal craniosynostosis include *FGFR2*, *FGFR3*, *TWIST1*, *EFNB1*, *ERF*, and *TCF12*.[3] In addition, Saethre–Chotzen (SCS) and Muenke syndrome, can present with this form of SSC.[3] Therefore, genetic consultation is recommended in all cases of unicoronal craniosynostosis. Please see additional details in the MSC section later in discussion.

Some additional management recommendations are associated with unicoronal craniosynostosis. Because 50% to 65% of patients with unicoronal craniosynostosis develop strabismus from the distortion in orbital shape and a resulting impact on the muscle insertions of extraocular muscles,[45,46] they should be evaluated by ophthalmology. There is a risk of persistent strabismus, amblyopia, and strabismus after surgical treatment.[47] Patients with unicoronal craniosynostosis also have an increased risk of an associated cervical spine anomaly, they should have spine imaging at the time of cranial vault imaging.[48,49]

Lambdoid craniosynostosis

Fusion of one lambdoid suture leads to flattening of the parietal and occipital bones on the affected side (**Fig. 6**). Because of growth restriction whereby the suture is fused, the mastoid process will become more prominent on the affected side and the skull base will appear to be tilted. The skull becomes distorted as the brain grows, resulting in prominence of the parietal skull on the unaffected side, often with a facial twist as growth continues whereby sutures are patent. The ear on the affected side often is lower than the opposite ear because of growth restriction on the affected side. The ear position in the horizontal position is more variable but can be posterior to the ear on the unaffected side.

The overall head shapes of unilateral coronal and lambdoid craniosynostoses are sometimes referred to as anterior and posterior plagiocephaly, respectively. This can create confusion, however, because the term "plagiocephaly" generally refers to positional plagiocephaly, which has become very common over the past 3 decades as the initiation of the Back to Sleep campaign in 1992.[50,51] The differentiation between positional plagiocephaly and unilateral lambdoid craniosynostosis is an important and common task for any provider assessing head shape concerns. In the case of positional plagiocephaly, there is no restriction of growth, as all sutures are open. Therefore, there is no mastoid bulge on the flattened side, and the skull base remains level. If there is flattening of the forehead, it should be of the contralateral side from the parieto-occipital flattening. Ear position should not be affected in the vertical plane, but the ear ipsilateral to the flattening may be pushed anterior to the other ear in the horizontal plane.[52]

Lambdoid craniosynostosis is the rarest form of SSC, occurring in < less than 1 per 10,000 live births.[15,16] It affects men more often than women in a 3:1 ratio.[16] Unilateral lambdoid craniosynostosis carries a significant risk for Chiari malformations, including 60% in one recent study.[53] An

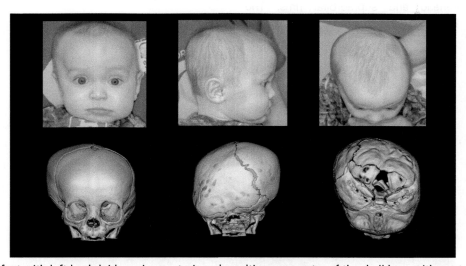

Fig. 6. Infant with left lambdoid craniosynostosis and resulting asymmetry of the skull base with mastoid bulge and facial asymmetry.

MRI to evaluate for cerebellar tonsil herniation should be performed as part of the presurgical work-up, as its presence can have an impact on the surgical approach that will reduce the risk of a symptomatic Chiari malformation in the future.[53]

IMAGING

Figs. 2–6 depict the head shapes of infants with the SSC described above. It is important to note that there can be cases that are subtle. Perception of a ridge along a suture can be concerning for craniosynostosis, but it can also be misleading. In some cases, neuroimaging is required to confirm a clinical diagnosis. Some centers may offer ultrasound of cranial sutures with skilled technicians, and CT scan is also recommended to confirm the diagnosis and for surgical planning. Diagnosis of metopic craniosynostosis can be particularly challenging when the trigonocephaly is mild, because the metopic suture normally fuses during infancy, somewhere between 3 and 9 months of age.[44] The other major sutures typically fuse in adulthood, likely in the second or third decade,[1] although there is some emerging evidence for earlier closure of the sagittal suture.[54]

Multi-suture craniosynostosis

MSC is defined as having coexisting anomalies associated with fused cranial sutures, often occurring in areas that are distinct from the skull. Patients with MSC often have more than one suture close prematurely, and several genetic variants are associated with MSC. Fig. 7 shows an infant with bicoronal craniosynostosis, illustrating brachycephaly and turricephaly with bilateral retruded forehead and supraorbital rims. The management of patients with MSC is more complex, as they are more likely to need intervention not only to expand the cranial vault, but also to treat upper airway obstruction, malocclusion, and often problems with vision, hearing, and speech. These patients are best managed by a multidisciplinary team with expertise in the management of children with complex craniofacial conditions.

Although there are numerous types of MSC, and all of these are far less common than SSC, there are 5 syndromes that are most commonly seen among cases of MSC (Table 1). Crouzon, caused by various mutations in fibroblast growth factor receptor type 2 (FGFR2), is autosomal dominant and quite variable in the range of severity. Most patients with Crouzon have brachycephaly, often from bicoronal craniosynostosis, with associated midface hypoplasia and malocclusion. Apert syndrome is also caused by mutations in specific regions of FGFR2. In addition to head shape differences from the fusion of multiple sutures, patients with Apert syndrome often have symmetric syndactyly of hands and feet, as well as a beaked nose. Pfeiffer syndrome, caused by mutations in FGFR1 or FGFR2, is subdivided into several types, some of which are associated with kleeblattschadel, or clover leaf skull, which is the most severe form of MSC. Patients with Pfeiffer syndrome often have tracheal sleeve or other tracheal anomalies, joint fusion of upper or lower extremities, and broad thumbs and great toes, sometimes with partial soft-tissue syndactyly. SCS, associated with mutations in TWIST1, is autosomal dominant and may have less severe presentation relative to the others. Patients with SCS often have low anterior hairline, eyelid ptosis, and prominent crus or other

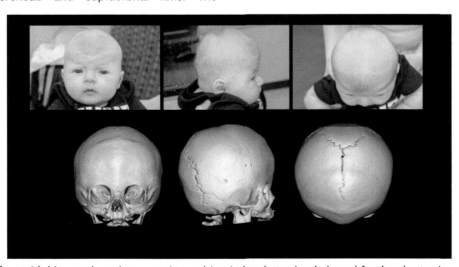

Fig. 7. Infant with bicoronal craniosynostosis, resulting in brachyturricephaly and forehead retrusion.

Table 1
Most common syndromic forms of craniosynostosis are outlined, including name of syndrome, gene, and inheritance pattern

Syndrome	Gene	Inheritance	Craniofacial Phenotype	Associated Anomalies	Cognition
Crouzon	*FGFR2*	Autosomal dominant; often de novo	Craniosynostosis with consequent head shape abnormalities (often brachycephaly); shallow orbits with ocular proptosis; high-arched palate; midface hypoplasia; anterior open bite	Hearing loss; variable respiratory issues (choanal stenosis, tongue-based obstruction, tracheal); Chiari I malformation; hydrocephalus; cervical spine fusion	Normal or near normal
Apert	*FGFR2*	Autosomal dominant; often de novo	Turribrachycephaly due to multi-suture craniosynostosis; shallow orbits with ocular proptosis; mild hypertelorism; down-slanting palpebral fissures; high-arched or cleft palate; severe midface hypoplasia; anterior open bite; "parrot beak" nasal deformity	Hearing loss; Symmetric syndactyly of hands and feet (often fusion of second, third, and fourth fingers/toes); synostosis of radius and humerus; multilevel airway obstruction common (choanal stenosis, tongue-based, tracheal); malrotation; hyperhidrosis; acne; fused cervical vertebrae; cardiac anomalies	Significantly increased incidence of intellectual disability
Pfeiffer	*FGFR2* *FGFR1*	Autosomal dominant; often de novo	Type I (classic): turribrachycephaly; midface hypoplasia; ocular proptosis, hypertelorism, strabismus, down-slanting palpebral fissures; beaked nasal deformity; anterior open bite Type II: kleeblattschadel; severe ocular proptosis Type III: kleeblattschadel; severe ocular proptosis; marked shortening of anterior cranial base	Hearing loss; broad thumbs and great toes; partial soft-tissue syndactyly of hands; multilevel airway obstruction (choanal atresia/stenosis, tongue-based, tracheal anomalies including tracheal sleeve; synostosis of radius and humerus, knee ankylosis)	Normal to significant intellectual disability

(continued on next page)

Table 1 *(continued)*

Syndrome	Gene	Inheritance	Craniofacial Phenotype	Associated Anomalies	Cognition
Muenke	*FGFR3*	Autosomal dominant (incomplete penetrance); can be de novo	Craniosynostosis of coronal sutures; variable degree of midface retrusion; hypertelorism	Hearing loss; variable skeletal differences: thimble-like middle phalanges, brachydactyly, carpal, and tarsal bone fusions, coned epiphyses	Normal to mild intellectual disability; ADHD; seizures
Saethre-Chotzen	*TWIST1*	Autosomal dominant; often de novo	Heterogeneous patterns of craniosynostosis; low frontal hairline; eyelid ptosis; facial asymmetry; deviated nasal septum; ear deformities with prominent crus helices extending through conchal bowl	Hearing loss; brachydactyly, broad toes, partial soft-tissue 2–3 syndactyly of hands	Normal to significant intellectual disability

Also included are craniofacial phenotype, associated anomalies, and expected cognition.

forms of dysplastic ears. Muenke syndrome may have physical characteristics that are more subtle and is therefore more difficult to diagnose. Muenke syndrome is autosomal dominant with incomplete penetrance and caused by mutations in *FGFR3*. Patients typically have unicoronal craniosynostosis, sometimes with midface retrusion or hypertelorism, and are also at risk for hearing loss and seizures. Management of patients with these syndromes is discussed in detail later in this volume.

CLINICS CARE POINTS

- Craniosynostosis can usually be diagnosed based on head shape, but a CT confirms the diagnosis and is used for surgical planning.
- Most benign head shape differences that may be confused with craniosynostosis improve with time, but abnormal head shapes associated with craniosynostosis will worsen as the child grows.
- Patients with unicoronal craniosynostosis should be offered genetic testing, but without additional medical concerns or associated malformations, genetic testing is lower yield for patients with SSC involving other sutures.
- Patients with craniosynostosis causing facial asymmetry (ie, unicoronal, lambdoid) should be referred for an ophthalmology evaluation to monitor alignment.

DISCLOSURE

The authors have nothing to disclose.

REFERENCES

1. Cohen MM, MacLean RE. Craniosynostosis : diagnosis, evaluation, and management. 2nd edition. New York: Oxford University Press. xx; 2000. p. 454.
2. Twigg SR, Wilkie AO. A Genetic-Pathophysiological Framework for Craniosynostosis. Am J Hum Genet 2015;97(3):359–77.
3. Wilkie AO, Johnson D, Wall SA. Clinical genetics of craniosynostosis. Curr Opin Pediatr 2017;29:622–8.
4. Lenton K, Nacamuli R, Wan D. Cranial suture biology. Curr Top Dev Biol 2005;66:287–328.
5. Renier D, Sainte-Rose C, Marchac D, et al. Intracranial pressure in craniostenosis. J Neurosurg 1982;57(3):370–7.
6. Gault DT, Renier D, Marchac D, et al. Intracranial pressure and intracranial volume in children with craniosynostosis. Plast Reconstr Surg 1992;90(3):377–81.
7. Pellicer E, Siebold BS, Birgfeld CB, et al. Evaluating Trends in Headache and Revision Surgery following Cranial Vault Remodeling for Craniosynostosis. Plast Reconstr Surg 2018;141(3):725–34.
8. Starr JR, Kapp-Simon KA, Cloonan YK, et al. Presurgical and postsurgical assessment of the neurodevelopment of infants with single-suture craniosynostosis: comparison with controls. J Neurosurg 2007;107(2 Suppl):103–10.
9. Starr JR, Collett BR, Gaither R, et al. Multicenter study of neurodevelopment in 3-year-old children with and without single-suture craniosynostosis. Arch Pediatr Adolesc Med 2012;166(6):536–42.
10. Speltz ML, Collett BR, Wallace ER, et al. Intellectual and academic functioning of school-age children with single-suture craniosynostosis. Pediatrics 2015;135(3):e615–23.
11. Kapp-Simon KA, Speltz ML, Cunningham ML, et al. Neurodevelopment of children with single suture craniosynostosis: a review. Childs Nerv Syst 2007;23:269–81.
12. Kapp-Simon KA, Wallace E, Collett BR, et al. Language, learning, and memory in children with and without single-suture craniosynostosis. J Neurosurg Pediatr 2016;17(5):578–88.
13. Schraw JM, Woodhouse JP, Langlois PH, et al. Risk factors and time trends for isolated craniosynostosis. Birth Defects Res 2021;113(1):43–54.
14. Lee HQ, et al. Changing Epidemiology of Nonsyndromic Craniosynostosis and Revisiting the Risk Factors. J Craniofac Surg 2012;23(5):1245–51.
15. Tønne E, Due-Tonnessen BJ, Wiig U, et al. Epidemiology of craniosynostosis in Norway. J Neurosurg Pediatr 2020;26(1):68–75.
16. Cornelissen M, Ottelander B, Rizopoulos D, et al. Increase of prevalence of craniosynostosis. J Craniomaxillofac Surg 2016;44(9):1273–9.
17. Abdelhamid K, Konci R, ElHawary H, et al. Advanced parental age: Is it contributing to an increased incidence of non-syndromic craniosynostosis? A review of case-control studies. J Oral Biol Craniofac Res 2021;11(1):78–83.
18. Carmichael SL, Ma C, Rasmussen SA, et al. Craniosynostosis and Maternal Smoking. Birth Defects Res (Part A) 2008;82:78–85.
19. Jentink J, Loane MA, Dolk H, et al. Valproic Acid Monotherapy in Pregnancy and Major Congenital Malformations. N Engl J Med 2010;362:2185–93.
20. Lajeunie E, Barcik U, Thorne JA, et al. Craniosynostosis and fetal exposure to sodium valproate. J Neurosurg 2001;95:778–82.
21. Singh RP, Dhariwal D, Bhujel N, et al. Role of parental risk factors in the aetiology of isolated non-syndromic metopic craniosynostosis. Br J Oral Maxillofacial Surg 2010;48:438–42.
22. Kallen B, Robert-Gnansia E. Maternal Drug Use, Fertility Problems, and Infant Craniostenosis. Cleft Palate Craniofac J 2005;42(6):589–93.
23. Goldberg O, Moretti M, Levy A, et al. Exposure to Nitrofurantoin During Early Pregnancy and Congenital

Malformations: A Systematic Review and Meta-Analysis. J Obstet Gynaecol Can 2015;37(2):150–6.

24. Berard A, Zhao JP, Sheehy O. Sertraline use during pregnancy and the risk of major malformations. Am J Obstet Gynecol 2015;212(6):795.e1-e12.

25. Louik C, Lin AE, Werler MM, et al. First-Trimester Use of Selective Serotonin-Reuptake Inhibitors and the Risk of Birth Defects. N Engl J Med 2007;356:2675–83.

26. Carmichael SL, Rasmussen SA, Lammer EJ, et al. Craniosynostosis and nutrient intake during pregnancy. Birth Defects Res A Clin Mol Teratol 2010;88(12):1032–9.

27. Rasmussen SA, Yazdy MM, Carmichael SL, et al. Maternal Thyroid Disease as a Risk Factor for Craniosynostosis. Obstet Gynecol 2007;110(2):369–77.

28. Carmichael SL, Ma C, Rasmussen SA, et al. Craniosynostosis and Risk Factors Related to Thyroid Dysfunction. Am J Med Genet 2015;0(4):701–7.

29. Akita S, Nakamura T, Hirano A, et al. Thyroid hormone action on rat calvarial sutures. Thyroid 1994;4:99–106.

30. Vega RA, Opalak C, Harshbarger RJ, et al. Hypophosphatemic rickets and craniosynostosis: a multicenter case series. J Neurosurg Pediatr 2016;17:694–700.

31. Di Rocco F, Rothenbuhler A, Cormier Daire V, et al. Craniosynostosis and metabolic bone disorder. A review. Neurosurgery 2019;65:258–63.

32. Cohen MM. Etiopathogenesis of craniosynostosis. Neurosurg Clin North America 1991;2(3):507–13.

33. Cohen MM. Sutural biology and the correlates of craniosynostosis. Am J Med Genet A 1993;47(5):581–616.

34. Bryant JR, Mantilla-Rivas E, Keating RF, et al. Craniosynostosis Develops in Half of Infants Treated for Hydrocephalus with a Ventriculoperitoneal Shunt. Plast Reconstr Surg 2021;147(6):1390–9.

35. Sanchez-Lara PA, Carmichael SL, Graham JM, et al. Fetal constraint as a potential risk factor for craniosynostosis. Am J Med Genet Part A 2010;152A(2):394–400.

36. Clarke CM, Fok VT, Gustafson JA, et al. Single suture craniosynostosis: Identification of rare variants in genes associated with syndromic forms. Am J Med Genet Part A 2018;176(2):290–300.

37. Boyadjiev SA. Genetic analysis of non-syndromic craniosynostosis. Orthod Craniofac Res 2007;10:129–37.

38. Justice CM, Yagnik G, Kim Y, et al. A genome-wide association study identifies susceptibility loci for nonsyndromic sagittal craniosynostosis near BMP2 and within BBS9. Nat Genet 2012;44(12):1360–4.

39. Greenwood J, Flodman P, Osann K, et al. Familial incidence and associated symptoms in a population of individuals with nonsyndromic craniosynostosis. Genet Med 2014;16(4):302–10.

40. Sacks GN, Skolnick GB, Trachtenberg A, et al. The Impact of Ethnicity on Craniosynostosis in the United States. J Craniofac Surg 2019;30(8):2526–9.

41. Anderson IA, Goomany A, Bonthron DT, et al. Does patient ethnicity affect site of craniosynostosis? J Neurosurg Pediatr 2014;14:682–7.

42. Gallagher ER, Evans KN, Hing AV, et al. Bathrocephaly: A Head Shape Associated With a Persistent Mendosal Suture. Cleft Palate Craniofac J 2013;50(1):104–8.

43. Birgfeld CB, Saltzman BS, Hing AV, et al. Making the diagnosis: metopic ridge versus metopic craniosynostosis. J Craniofac Surg 2013;24(1):178–85.

44. Weinzweig J, Kirschner RE, Farley A, et al. Metopic synostosis: Defining the temporal sequence of normal suture fusion and differentiating it from synostosis on the basis of computed tomography images. Plast Reconstr Surg 2003;112(5):1211–8.

45. Di Rocco C, Paternoster G, Caldarelli M, et al. Anterior plagiocephaly: epidemiology, clinical findings, diagnosis, and classification. A review. Child's Nervous Syst 2012;28(9):1413–22.

46. Macintosh C, Wall S, Leach C. Strabismus in unicoronal synostosis: ipsilateral or contralateral? J Craniofac Surg 2007;18(3):465–9.

47. MacKinnon S, Proctor MR, Rogers GF, et al. Improving ophthalmic outcomes in children with unilateral coronal synostosis by treatment with endoscopic strip craniectomy and helmet therapy rather than fronto-orbital advancement. J AAPOS 2013;17(3):259–65.

48. Kruszka, P., Addissie, Y.A., Agochukwu, N.B., et al., Muenke Syndrome, in GeneReviews((R)), M.P. Adam, et al., Editors. 1993: Seattle (WA).

49. Gallagher, E.R., C. Ratisoontorn, and M.L. Cunningham, Saethre-Chotzen Syndrome, in GeneReviews((R)), M.P. Adam, et al., Editors. 1993: Seattle (WA).

50. Kane AA, Mitchell LE, Craven KP, et al. Observations on a Recent Increase in Plagiocephaly Without Synostosis. Pediatrics 1996;97(6):877–85.

51. Mawji A, Vollman AR, Hatfield J, et al. The Incidence of Positional Plagiocephaly: A Cohort Study. Pediatrics 2013;132(2):298–304.

52. Huang MH, Mouradian WE, Cohen SR, et al. The differential diagnosis of abnormal head shapes: separating craniosynostosis from positional deformities and normal variants. Cleft Palate Craniofac J 1998;35(3):204–11.

53. Fearon JA, Dimas V, Ditthakasem K. Lambdoid Craniosynostosis: The Relationship with Chiari Deformations and an Analysis of Surgical Outcomes. Plast Reconstr Surg 2016;137(3):946–51.

54. Wilkinson CC, Stence NV, Serrano CA, et al. Fusion patterns of major calvarial sutures on volume-rendered CT reconstructions. J Neurosurg Pediatr 2020;25(5):519–28.

Multidisciplinary Care Considerations for Patients with Craniosynostosis

Emily R. Gallagher, MD[a,b,c,*], G. Kyle Fulton, MD[c],
Srinivas M. Susarla, DMD, MD, MPH[b], Craig B. Birgfeld, MD[b]

KEYWORDS

- Craniosynostosis • Multidisciplinary care • Craniofacial team

KEY POINTS

- Optimal care of patients with craniosynostosis requires coordinated, longitudinal multidisciplinary care.
- The craniofacial team is composed of specialists from a wide variety of disciplines, each of whom provide a critical contribution to the care of patients with craniosynostosis.
- Standardized clinical care pathways can help set expectations for patients and families, establish timelines for medical and surgical interventions, and allow the team to critically evaluate results over time.

INTRODUCTION

Craniosynostosis remains one of the most common congenital conditions seen in multidisciplinary craniofacial clinics.[1–9] The prevalence of the condition ranges from 3 to 5 cases per 10,000 births, with greater than 80% of affected patients having non-syndromic presentations.[1–4] Single-suture craniosynostosis encompasses the majority of cases, of which sagittal synostosis is the most common form.[2–5] Syndromic craniosynostosis is estimated to represent approximately 10% of cases and typically involves multiple sutures. There are more than 150 syndromes associated with craniosynostosis, with bicoronal synostosis the most common presentation of syndromic cases.[9–11] The epidemiology, pathophysiology, and genetics of craniosynostosis are discussed elsewhere in this volume.

Given the complexity of the condition, as well as the age at which patients are diagnosed and treated, multidisciplinary care is the standard for managing patients with craniosynostoses.[6–9] The multidisciplinary team consists of numerous specialists who work together to achieve a holistic, coordinated, safe, and efficacious treatment of patients from infancy through skeletal maturity and adulthood (**Fig. 1**). Although each specialist has a defined area of expertise, the collaborative model of patient care is most effective when specialists share their knowledge and skills. This article highlights the various members of the multidisciplinary team and their specific roles in the management of patients with craniosynostoses. Surgical care pathways for the various types of synostoses are discussed later.

CRANIOSYNOSTOSIS TEAM MEMBERS

Each multidisciplinary craniofacial team may consist of slightly different core or ancillary members but should have ready access to at least the

[a] Department of Pediatrics, Division of Craniofacial Medicine, University of Washington and Seattle Children's Hospital, 4800 Sand Point Way Northeast, M/S OB.9.520, PO Box 5371, Seattle, WA 98145-5005, USA; [b] Craniofacial Center, Seattle Children's Hospital, University of Washington, Seattle, WA, USA; [c] Louisiana State University School of Medicine, New Orleans, LA, USA
* Corresponding author. Department of Pediatrics, Division of Craniofacial Medicine, University of Washington and Seattle Children's Hospital, 4800 Sand Point Way Northeast, M/S OB.9.520, PO Box 5371, Seattle, WA 98145-5005.
E-mail address: emily.gallagher@seattlechildrens.org

Oral Maxillofacial Surg Clin N Am 34 (2022) 353–365
https://doi.org/10.1016/j.coms.2022.04.001
1042-3699/22/© 2022 Elsevier Inc. All rights reserved.

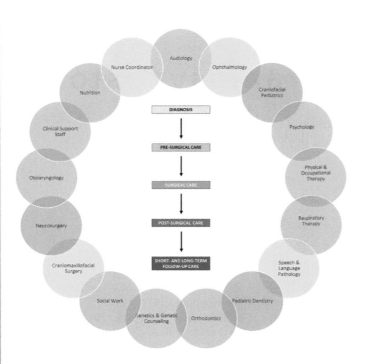

Fig. 1. Coordinated, multidisciplinary care is mandated for patients with single- and multi-suture craniosynostoses from diagnosis through long-term follow-up after intervention.

following specialists. One resource to find a local, accredited craniofacial team is the American Cleft Palate-Craniofacial Association Team Finder Web site.[12]

Clinical Support Staff

Coordinated care for patients with craniosynostosis requires a seamless coordination of scheduling to ensure efficient clinic visits while giving special attention to the specific needs of each patient. In this regard, clinical support staff have an integral role in the structure and function of the craniofacial team, ensuring that patients and families have an organized framework for care plans and contact points when questions arise.

Craniofacial Pediatrics

The craniofacial pediatrician is a critical team member who assesses medical, nutritional, and developmental health of the child and may serve as a liaison between outside primary care providers and the team. The craniofacial pediatricians are often the first point of contact for patients and families, consider broad aspects of the child's health, explain the diagnosis and plan of care, and bring in other subspecialty providers as needed. The craniofacial pediatrician has specific expertise in the diagnosis, management, and prognosis for patients with craniosynostosis as well as other associated issues or conditions.

They work with all team members to provide a holistic approach by managing medical issues related to their craniosynostosis, coordinating care across all specialties, and helping the team to provide a unified treatment plan for each patient. The craniofacial pediatricians also consider whether there may be an underlying genetic variant and can help facilitate genetic testing when appropriate.

Craniomaxillofacial Surgery

Craniomaxillofacial (CMF) surgeons play a key role in the management of patients with craniosynostosis. The CMF surgeon works with pediatric neurosurgery to map a surgical plan timed to optimize safety, brain growth and development, facial growth, physical appearance, and social adjustment. Typically, the first surgical intervention is in infancy for correction of skull constriction. Secondary procedures for cranial vault reconstruction or frontofacial procedures may be necessary later in childhood. As children enter mixed dentition, subcranial surgery may be indicated to address midface hypoplasia, orbital dystopia, or other facial anomalies. At skeletal maturity, many patients with craniosynostosis will have end-stage maxillomandibular discrepancies that are corrected with orthognathic approaches.

In addition, surgeons may provide guidance or surgical interventions for other associated conditions, seen in patients with syndromic

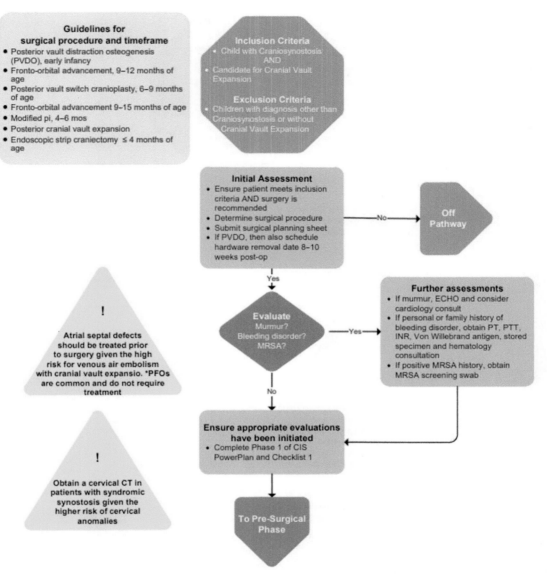

Fig. 2. Diagnostic phase. (*From* Seattle Children's Hospital, Birgfeld C, Heike C, Herrman A, Popalisky J, Turner A. March 2019. Craniosynostosis Pathway. http://www.seattlechildrens.org/pdf/craniosynostosis-pathway.pdf.)

craniosynostosis, such as syndactyly in patients with Apert syndrome.

Pediatric Neurosurgery

Neurosurgical care is necessary in patients with craniosynostosis and some commonly associated conditions. Neurosurgeons provide expertise and assure patient safety when discussing or performing primary interventions to manage cephalocranial disproportion requiring craniotomies for bony expansion and reshaping or other frontofacial procedures that include the skull base and orbits. Patients with syndromic craniosynostoses are at

higher risk of having neurologic conditions that need surgical monitoring or management: cervical spine abnormalities, hydrocephalus, or Arnold–Chiari malformations.

Nurse Coordinator

Nurse coordinators maintain the relationship and facilitate communication between the medical team and families and often serve as the single contact person for a family throughout the continuum of care. They frequently provide the patient and family with education to prepare them for surgery, as well as understand and demonstrate the

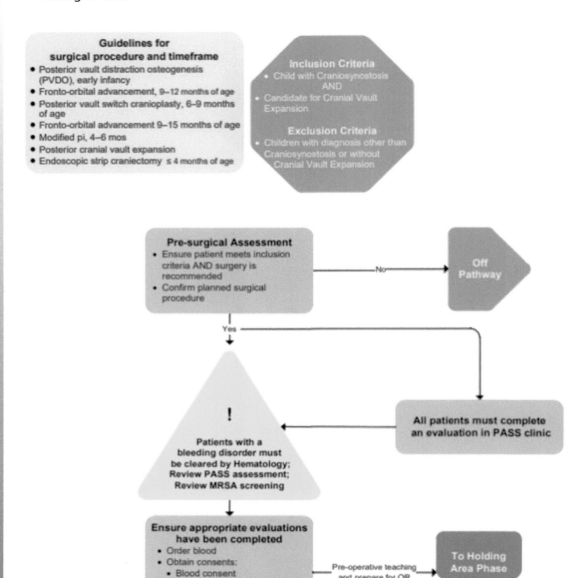

Fig. 3. Presurgical phase. (*From* Seattle Children's Hospital, Birgfeld C, Heike C, Herrman A, Popalisky J, Turner A. March 2019. Craniosynostosis Pathway. http://www.seattlechildrens.org/pdf/craniosynostosis-pathway.pdf.)

care needed after surgery. Nurse coordinators help the family understand the current state of care, track progress, and anticipating future challenges they may face.

Otolaryngology

One of the most emergent issues facing infants with craniosynostosis is an upper airway obstruction or other airway anomalies, particularly in those with syndromic synostosis.[13] This can be caused by facial skeletal dysmorphology (eg, midface hypoplasia) or primary airway anomalies (eg, laryngomalacia, tracheomalacia, cartilaginous sleeves).[14,15] The otolaryngologist serves a fundamental role on the craniofacial team in the initial evaluation and management of upper airway obstruction. Their continual involvement is essential to ensure airway safety, particularly in patients undergoing sequential interventions under general anesthesia or surgeries involving

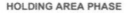

HOLDING AREA PHASE

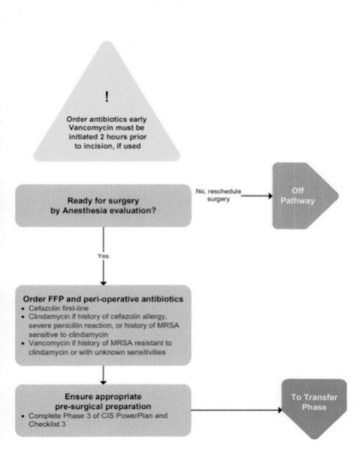

Fig. 4. Immediate preoperative care. (*From* Seattle Children's Hospital, Birgfeld C, Heike C, Herrman A, Popalisky J, Turner A. March 2019. Craniosynostosis Pathway. http://www.seattlechildrens.org/pdf/craniosynostosis-pathway.pdf.)

the maxilla and mandible. Otolaryngologists collaborate with audiology to evaluate and manage hearing loss.

Some patients with syndromic craniosynostosis can have severe, multilevel upper airway obstruction requiring immediate intervention at birth.[14] When syndromic craniosynostosis is suspected prenatally, otolaryngology should be involved in planning of the delivery to provide a secure airway.

Audiology

Patients with craniosynostosis are at higher risk of having hearing loss.[16,17] Untreated hearing loss can lead to difficulties in speech and language development, social-emotional development, and negatively impact learning. Audiologists are crucial to identifying, monitoring, and treating hearing loss throughout a patient's lifetime.

Genetics and Genetic Counseling

Geneticists and genetic counselors may help to identify a unifying genetic etiology in the children

with syndromic craniosynostosis by guiding genetic testing. Several genetic mutations may share a clinical phenotype on presentation, but have differing associated conditions, need for screening evaluations, or prognosis. This information is invaluable when crafting individual treatment plans for a patient. The genetics team also counsels the family on potential inheritance for future sibling or offspring of the patient.

Pediatric Dentistry

Pediatric dentists monitor oral hygiene and encourage positive dental habits at an early age. Many patients with craniosynostosis will have associated dentofacial differences: disturbances in tooth development, eruption, or discrepancies in jaw size.[18] They provide preventative and restorative dental care. Odontogenic infections can be challenging to manage in patients with craniosynostosis, particularly in those with other medical conditions, such as upper airway obstruction or shunted hydrocephalus. A longitudinal

PICU TRANSFER AND
SURGICAL UNIT TRANSFER PHASES

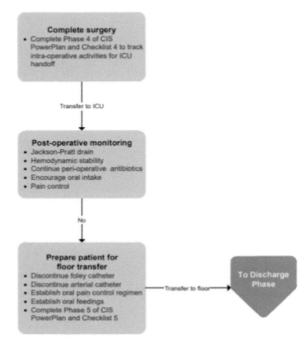

Continue peri-operative antibiotics
- Cefazolin first-line
- Clindamycin if history of cefazolin allergy, severe penicillin reaction, or history of MRSA sensitive to clindamycin
- Vancomycin if history of MRSA resistant to clindamycin or with unknown sensitivities

Complete surgery
- Complete Phase 4 of CIS PowerPlan and Checklist 4 to track intra-operative activities for ICU handoff

Transfer to ICU

Post-operative monitoring
- Jackson-Pratt drain
- Hemodynamic stability
- Continue peri-operative antibiotics
- Encourage oral intake
- Pain control

No

Prepare patient for floor transfer
- Discontinue foley catheter
- Discontinue arterial catheter
- Establish oral pain control regimen
- Establish oral feedings
- Complete Phase 5 of CIS PowerPlan and Checklist 5

Transfer to floor

To Discharge Phase

Fig. 5. Inpatient care. (*From* Seattle Children's Hospital, Birgfeld C, Heike C, Herrman A, Popalisky J, Turner A. March 2019. Craniosynostosis Pathway. http://www.seattlechildrens.org/pdf/craniosynostosis-pathway.pdf.)

assessment of dental development and eruption, in conjunction with orthodontic care, is paramount for the preservation of teeth and achieving a functional occlusion.

Orthodontics

Craniofacial orthodontists play an integral role in longitudinal care for the patient with craniosynostosis. Although orthodontic treatment is typically initiated in late mixed dentition, it is essential to collaborate with orthodontists earlier for patients where frontofacial or subcranial surgery is considered as an early intervention. Osteotomies of the midface involving the late primary or early mixed dentition can have profound effects on development and eruption of the succedaneous teeth.[18] Owing to this, craniofacial orthodontists are key partners to surgeons when planning these interventions. As children transition into adult dentition, many will have end-stage dentofacial and occlusal differences that can be improved with orthodontic treatment; some may need orthognathic surgery where again the orthodontist plays a critical role in surgical planning and final arch coordination.

Speech and Language Pathology

Speech and language pathologists are vital in evaluating and treating difficulties with speech and feeding. Anatomic or physiologic differences seen in patients with craniosynostosis may contribute to feeding difficulties, speech delays, or difficulties with language skills.[19] Feeding therapy can help infants feed more effectively and is especially beneficial in babies with syndromic craniosynostosis and upper airway obstruction. Frequent monitoring for speech and language delays coupled with early intervention for identified or suspected delays helps ensure appropriate development throughout infancy into adulthood.

DISCHARGE PHASE

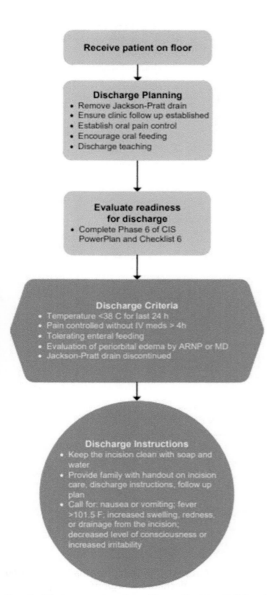

Fig. 6. Discharge planning. (*From* Seattle Children's Hospital, Birgfeld C, Heike C, Herrman A, Popalisky J, Turner A. March 2019. Craniosynostosis Pathway. http://www.seattlechildrens.org/pdf/craniosynostosis-pathway.pdf.)

Social Work

Social workers remain a cornerstone of the multidisciplinary team. Patients with craniosynostosis require extensive medical and surgical care with longitudinal multidisciplinary follow-up. The cumulative medical, mental, and financial burden that this entails can be immense and, at times, overwhelming for children and families. Social workers play a vital role with families to identify, prevent, and overcome barriers to care. They offer support and local resources for families that may include organizing or assistance with travel and lodging needed to receive care, facilitating support groups for families, or coordinating care for children that need specialized day-to-day or in-home care.

Respiratory Therapy

As with otolaryngologists, respiratory therapists are integral to the management of airway conditions in patients with craniosynostosis. Respiratory therapy involvement varies depending on a patient's airway anomalies or degree of obstruction and is not limited to the postoperative course. Some upper airway obstruction is treated with noninvasive methods (eg, CPAP), while others may require tracheostomy placement as seen in severe multilevel obstruction. Input from respiratory therapists can help ensure safe care for patients with complex airway morphologies and may help avoid respiratory and pulmonary complications.

Ophthalmology

Ophthalmologic evaluation is important, as craniosynostosis can affect the functioning of the eyes in multiple ways. Patients with anterior cranial vault abnormalities may have orbital deformities with associated alterations in globe position or eye alignment.[20] Ophthalmologists provide treatment of these findings like tarsorrhaphy for corneal exposure or globe subluxation and extraocular muscle-balancing surgery for strabismus. In addition, cephalocranial disproportion can result in elevated intracranial pressure, which may be identified as papilledema on fundoscopic examination before the presentation of other clinical signs or symptoms. A frequent evaluation by ophthalmology, at least annually through childhood, is essential to ensure that subtle findings of elevated intracranial pressure or other visual anomalies are not missed. Advances in imaging modalities used by ophthalmology, like optical coherence tomography used to assess optic nerve function, will likely become more common place in the future and may help guide decisions about the appropriate type and timing of surgical treatments.[21]

Nutrition

A dietician with knowledge and experience with the specific challenges encountered in patients with craniosynostosis is essential to the craniofacial team to ensure continued adequate growth,

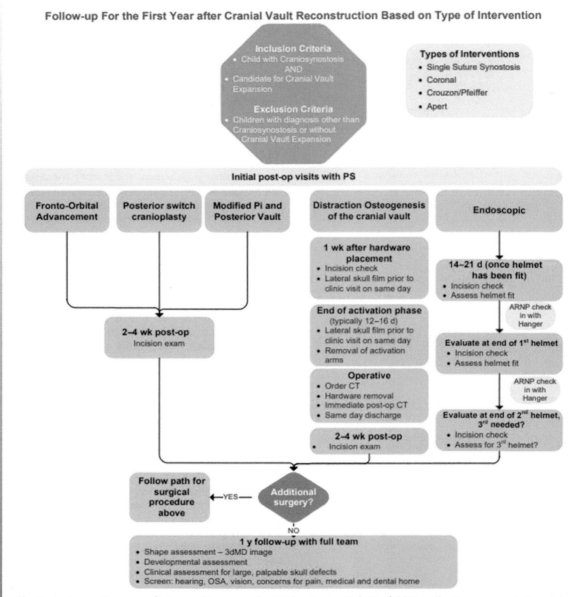

Fig. 7. Postoperative care—first year. (*From* Seattle Children's Hospital, Birgfeld C, Heike C, Herrman A, Popalisky J, Turner A. March 2019. Craniosynostosis Pathway. http://www.seattlechildrens.org/pdf/craniosynostosis-pathway.pdf.)

development, and post-op healing. Many children with craniosynostosis will undergo significant surgical interventions throughout life—optimal nutritional status is critical to ensure bony and soft tissue healing. Patients with syndromic craniosynostosis may require enteral feeding via gastrostomy tubes; requiring even closer monitoring of nutritional status and guidance of when/how to augment feeds. A nutritionist can also help a patient and family anticipate and prepare for

postoperative diet modifications that are typical after orthognathic surgery.

Psychology

Although there remains significant debate regarding the long-term cognitive outcomes in the surgical treatment of craniosynostosis,[23–26] ongoing neuropsychological assessment is necessary for patients with craniosynostosis.

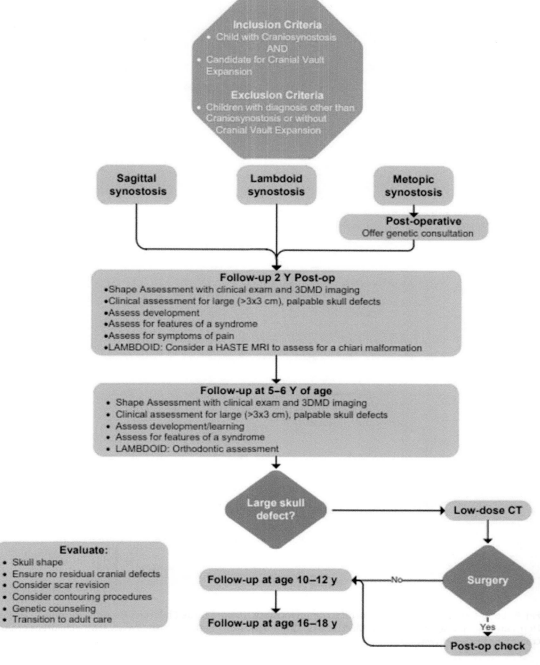

Fig. 8. Long-term follow-up care—sagittal, metopic, or lambdoid craniosynostosis. (*From* Seattle Children's Hospital, Birgfeld C, Heike C, Herrman A, Popalisky J, Turner A. March 2019. Craniosynostosis Pathway. http://www.seattlechildrens.org/pdf/craniosynostosis-pathway.pdf.)

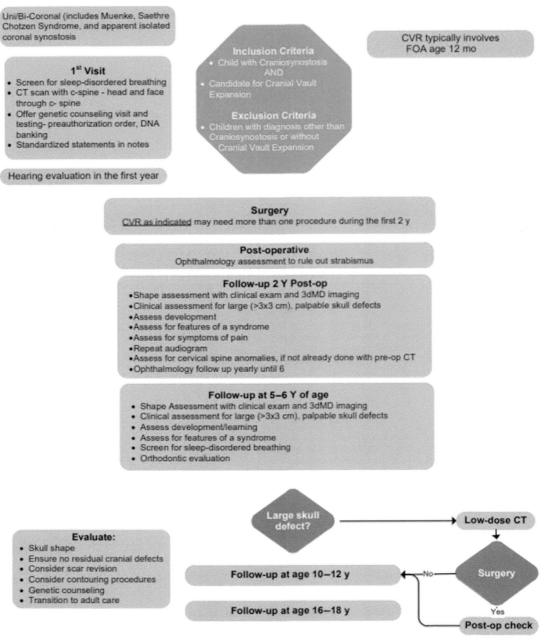

Fig. 9. Long-term follow-up care—coronal craniosynostosis. (*From* Seattle Children's Hospital, Birgfeld C, Heike C, Herrman A, Popalisky J, Turner A. March 2019. Craniosynostosis Pathway. http://www.seattlechildrens.org/pdf/craniosynostosis-pathway.pdf.)

This includes educational and learning evaluations performed by psychology before enrolling in school to give recommendations on how to best bolster the child's learning. Psychologists also play an invaluable role in helping children and adolescents cope with having craniofacial or other physical differences from their peers.

Occupational and Physical Therapy

Children with craniosynostosis are at higher risk of having developmental delays effecting mobility, coordination, and other gross and fine motor abilities. These can be compounded by associated neurologic conditions, ocular issues, syndactyly,

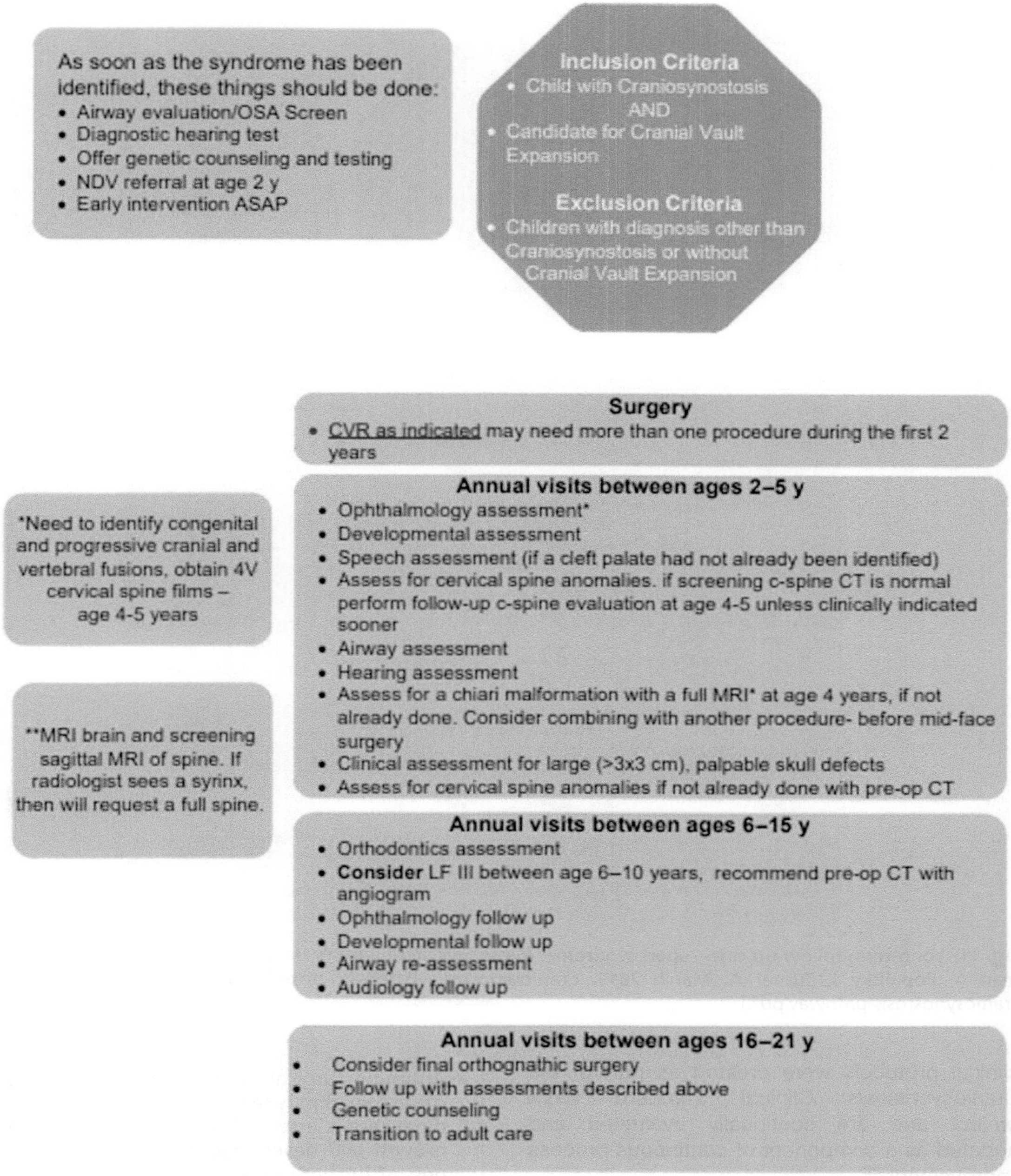

As soon as the syndrome has been identified, these things should be done:
- Airway evaluation/OSA Screen
- Diagnostic hearing test
- Offer genetic counseling and testing
- NDV referral at age 2 y
- Early intervention ASAP

Inclusion Criteria
- Child with Craniosynostosis AND
- Candidate for Cranial Vault Expansion

Exclusion Criteria
- Children with diagnosis other than Craniosynostosis or without Cranial Vault Expansion

Surgery
- CVR as indicated may need more than one procedure during the first 2 years

Annual visits between ages 2–5 y
- Ophthalmology assessment*
- Developmental assessment
- Speech assessment (if a cleft palate had not already been identified)
- Assess for cervical spine anomalies. if screening c-spine CT is normal perform follow-up c-spine evaluation at age 4-5 unless clinically indicated sooner
- Airway assessment
- Hearing assessment
- Assess for a chiari malformation with a full MRI* at age 4 years, if not already done. Consider combining with another procedure- before mid-face surgery
- Clinical assessment for large (>3x3 cm), palpable skull defects
- Assess for cervical spine anomalies if not already done with pre-op CT

*Need to identify congenital and progressive cranial and vertebral fusions, obtain 4V cervical spine films – age 4-5 years

**MRI brain and screening sagittal MRI of spine. If radiologist sees a syrinx, then will request a full spine.

Annual visits between ages 6–15 y
- Orthodontics assessment
- **Consider** LF III between age 6–10 years, recommend pre-op CT with angiogram
- Ophthalmology follow up
- Developmental follow up
- Airway re-assessment
- Audiology follow up

Annual visits between ages 16–21 y
- Consider final orthognathic surgery
- Follow up with assessments described above
- Genetic counseling
- Transition to adult care

Fig. 10. Long-term follow-up care—crouzon/pfeiffer syndrome. (*From* Seattle Children's Hospital, Birgfeld C, Heike C, Herrman A, Popalisky J, Turner A. March 2019. Craniosynostosis Pathway. http://www.seattlechildrens.org/pdf/craniosynostosis-pathway.pdf.)

needed medical technology (eg, gastrostomy tube or tracheostomy), and deconditioning from needed operations. Early evaluation and treatment by physical and occupational therapists can help improve the patient's overall developmental potential, speed recovery, and greatly improve quality of life.

COMPREHENSIVE CLINICAL CARE PATHWAY

Coordination between the care providers listed above can result in an efficient model of longitudinal care for patients with craniosynostosis. The model used at Seattle Children's Hospital institution is demonstrated in **Figs. 2–11**.[22] These

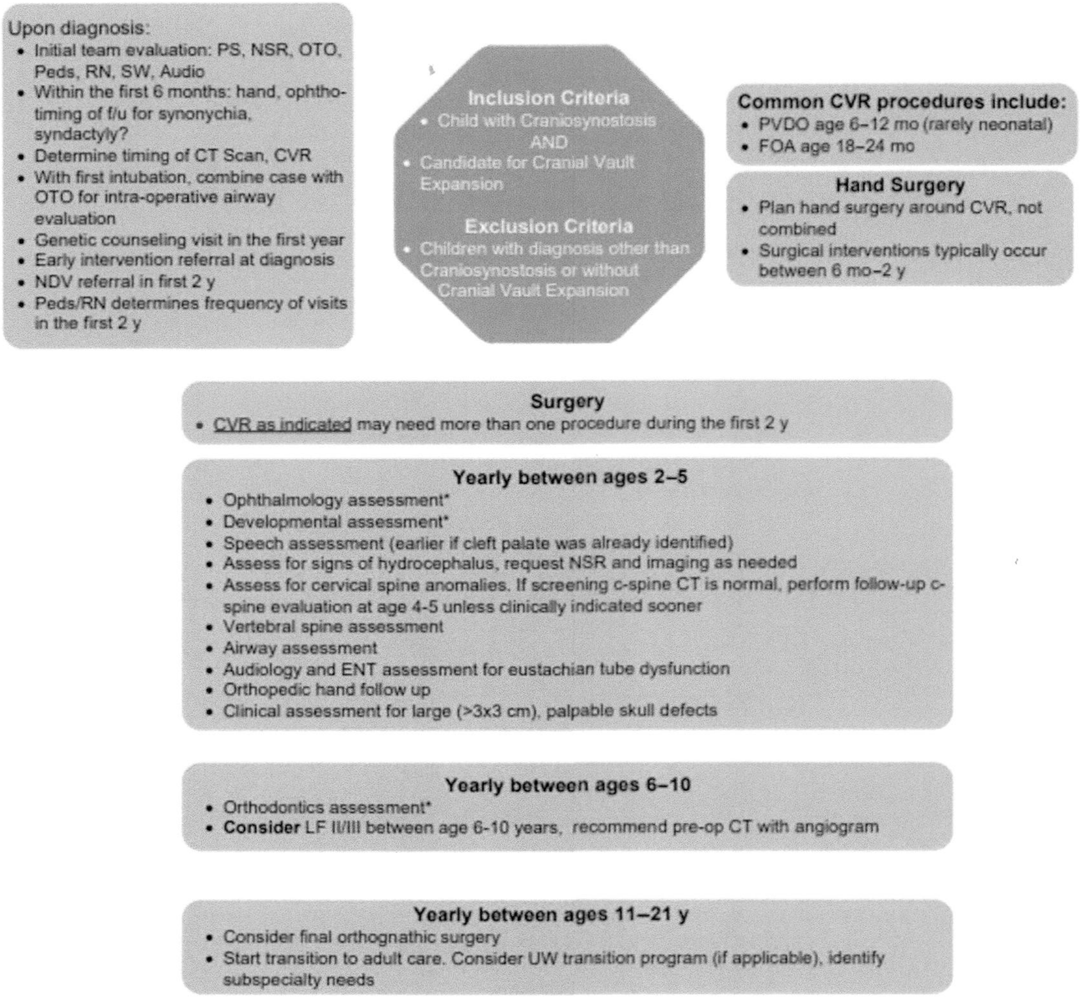

Upon diagnosis:
- Initial team evaluation: PS, NSR, OTO, Peds, RN, SW, Audio
- Within the first 6 months: hand, ophtho-timing of f/u for synonychia, syndactyly?
- Determine timing of CT Scan, CVR
- With first intubation, combine case with OTO for intra-operative airway evaluation
- Genetic counseling visit in the first year
- Early intervention referral at diagnosis
- NDV referral in first 2 y
- Peds/RN determines frequency of visits in the first 2 y

Inclusion Criteria
- Child with Craniosynostosis AND
- Candidate for Cranial Vault Expansion

Exclusion Criteria
- Children with diagnosis other than Craniosynostosis or without Cranial Vault Expansion

Common CVR procedures include:
- PVDO age 6–12 mo (rarely neonatal)
- FOA age 18–24 mo

Hand Surgery
- Plan hand surgery around CVR, not combined
- Surgical interventions typically occur between 6 mo–2 y

Surgery
- CVR as indicated may need more than one procedure during the first 2 y

Yearly between ages 2–5
- Ophthalmology assessment*
- Developmental assessment*
- Speech assessment (earlier if cleft palate was already identified)
- Assess for signs of hydrocephalus, request NSR and imaging as needed
- Assess for cervical spine anomalies. If screening c-spine CT is normal, perform follow-up c-spine evaluation at age 4-5 unless clinically indicated sooner
- Vertebral spine assessment
- Airway assessment
- Audiology and ENT assessment for eustachian tube dysfunction
- Orthopedic hand follow up
- Clinical assessment for large (>3x3 cm), palpable skull defects

Yearly between ages 6–10
- Orthodontics assessment*
- **Consider** LF II/III between age 6-10 years, recommend pre-op CT with angiogram

Yearly between ages 11–21 y
- Consider final orthognathic surgery
- Start transition to adult care. Consider UW transition program (if applicable), identify subspecialty needs

Fig. 11. Long-term follow-up care—apert syndrome. (*From* Seattle Children's Hospital, Birgfeld C, Heike C, Herrman A, Popalisky J, Turner A. March 2019. Craniosynostosis Pathway. http://www.seattlechildrens.org/pdf/craniosynostosis-pathway.pdf.)

clinical protocols were created as part of the Craniosynostosis Clinical Standard Work project and are continually evaluated and updated as a component of continuous process improvement.[22]

- Although surgical intervention in infancy is often the primary reason for referral, longitudinal care is essential to ensure appropriate growth and development as well as timeliness of further interventions as indicated.

CLINICS CARE POINTS

- The craniofacial team includes medical and surgical specialists who each bring an important perspective and clinical contribution to the care of patients with craniosynostosis

DISCLOSURE

The authors have no financial or non-financial interests related to this work.

REFERENCES

1. French LR, Jackson IT, Melton LJ 3rd. A population-based study of craniosynostosis. J Clin Epidemiol 1990;43(1):69–73.

2. Singer S, Bower C, Southall P, et al. Craniosynostosis in Western Australia, 1980-1994: a population-based study. Am J Med Genet 1999;83(5):382–7.

3. Boulet SL, Rasmussen SA, Honein MA. A population-based study of craniosynostosis in metropolitan Atlanta, 1989-2003. Am J Med Genet A 2008;146A(8):984–91.

4. Taylor JA, Bartlett SP. What's new in syndromic craniosynostosis surgery? Plast Reconstr Surg 2017; 140(1):82e–93e.

5. Garrocho-Rangel A, Manriquez-Olmos L, Flores-Velazquez J, et al. Non-syndromic craniosynostosis in children: Scoping review. Med Oral Patol Oral Cir Bucal 2018;23(4):e421–8.

6. Tahiri Y, Bartlett SP, Gilardino MS. Evidence-based medicine: nonsyndromic craniosynostosis. Plast Reconstr Surg 2017;140(1):177e–91e.

7. Chim H, Gosain AK. An evidence-based approach to craniosynostosis. Plast Reconstr Surg 2011; 127(2):910–7.

8. Birgfeld CB, Dufton L, Naumann H, et al. Safety of open cranial vault surgery for single-suture craniosynostosis: a case for the multidisciplinary team. J Craniofac Surg 2015;26(7):2052–8.

9. Buchanan EP, Xue Y, Xue AS, et al. Multidisciplinary care of craniosynostosis. J Multidiscip Healthc 2017; 10:263–70.

10. Rasmussen SA, Olney RS, Holmes LB, et al. Guidelines for case classification for the National Birth Defects Prevention Study. Birth Defects Res A Clin Mol Teratol 2003;67(3):193–201.

11. Cohen MM Jr. Craniosynostoses: phenotypic/molecular correlations. Am J Med Genet 1995;56(3):334–9.

12. American Cleft Palate-Craniofacial Association. Find a Team. ACPA. Available at: https://acpa-cpf.org/acpa-family-services/find-a-team/. Accessed March 11, 2022.

13. Mathews F, Shaffer AD, Georg MW, et al. Airway anomalies in patients with craniosynostosis. Laryngoscope 2019;129(11):2594–602.

14. Mathews F, Shaffer AD, Georg MW, et al. Laryngomalacia in patients with craniosynostosis. Ann Otol Rhinol Laryngol 2018;127(8):543–50.

15. Pickrell BB, Meaike JD, Cañadas KT, et al. Tracheal cartilaginous sleeve in syndromic craniosynostosis: an underrecognized source of significant morbidity and mortality. J Craniofac Surg 2017;28(3):696–9.

16. Agochukwu NB, Solomon BD, Muenke M. Hearing loss in syndromic craniosynostoses: otologic manifestations and clinical findings. Int J Pediatr Otorhinolaryngol 2014;78(12):2037–47.

17. Biamino E, Canale A, Lacilla M, et al. Prevention and management of hearing loss in syndromic craniosynostosis: A case series. Int J Pediatr Otorhinolaryngol 2016;85:95–8.

18. Vargervik K, Rubin MS, Grayson BH, et al. Parameters of care for craniosynostosis: dental and orthodontic perspectives. Am J Orthod Dentofacial Orthop 2012;141(4 Suppl):S68–73.

19. Kilcoyne S, Rajan SM, Dalton L, et al. The sensitivity and specificity of parental report of concern for identifying language disorder in children with craniosynostosis. J Craniofac Surg 2021;32(1):36–41.

20. Touzé R, Bremond-Gignac D, Robert MP. Ophthalmological management in craniosynostosis. Neurochirurgie 2019;65(5):310–7.

21. Kalmar CL, Humphries LS, McGeehan B, et al. Elevated intracranial pressure in patients with craniosynostosis by optical coherence tomography. Plast Reconstr Surg 2022;149(3): 677–90.

22. Seattle Children's Hospital, Birgfeld C, Heike C, Herrman A, et al. Craniosynostosis Pathway. 2019. Available at: http://www.seattlechildrens.org/pdf/craniosynostosis-pathway.pdf.

23. Mandela R, Bellew M, Chumas P, et al. Impact of surgery timing for craniosynostosis on neurodevelopmental outcomes: a systematic review. J Neurosurg Pediatr 2019;23(4):442–54. https://doi.org/10.3171/2018.10.PEDS18536.

24. Osborn AJ, Roberts RM, Mathias JL, et al. Cognitive, behavioral and psychological functioning in children with metopic synostosis: a meta-analysis examining the impact of surgical status. Child Neuropsychol 2019;25(2):263–77. https://doi.org/10.1080/09297049.2018.1441821.

25. Osborn AJ, Roberts RM, Dorstyn DS, et al. Sagittal synostosis and its association with cognitive, behavioral, and psychological functioning: a meta-analysis. JAMA Netw Open 2021;4(9):e2121937. https://doi.org/10.1001/jamanetworkopen.2021.21937. Published 2021 Sep 1.

26. Shim KW, Park EK, Kim JS, et al. Neurodevelopmental problems in non-syndromic craniosynostosis. J Korean Neurosurg Soc 2016;59(3):242–6. https://doi.org/10.3340/jkns.2016.59.3.242.

Fronto-Orbital Advancement for Metopic and Unilateral Coronal Craniosynostoses

Benjamin B. Massenburg, MD, Philip D. Tolley, MD, Amy Lee, MD, FAANS, Srinivas M. Susarla, DMD, MD, MPH*

KEYWORDS

- Metopic synostosis • Unicoronal synostosis • Unilateral coronal synostosis
- Fronto-orbital advancement • Anterior cranial vault reconstruction • Craniosynostosis

KEY POINTS

- Metopic craniosynostosis is characterized by a trigonocephalic head shape with lateral orbital retrusion and hypotelorism.
- Unilateral coronal craniosynostosis is characterized by ipsilateral retrusion of the forehead and an affected orbit that is taller and narrower (Harlequin deformity) than the unaffected side, which may have compensatory frontal bossing.
- Fronto-orbital advancement (FOA) is an effective treatment of the cranio-orbital deformities seen in metopic and unilateral craniosynostoses.
- Technical considerations for performing FOA in metopic and unilateral coronal synostosis include specific modifications to address the primary deformity and overcorrection to compensate for future growth and in the anticipation of relapse.

INTRODUCTION

Functional cranial sutures are critical in childhood, as they allow the expansion of the bony cranium for rapid brain growth and development. Bony deposition occurs as the skull expands perpendicular to each suture, and premature fusion of these sutures is known as craniosynostosis. In 1851, Virchow noted that a fused suture inhibits skull growth perpendicular to the direction of that suture, leading to compensatory growth at the remaining open sutures and resulting in cranial and skull base deformities.[1,2] Craniosynostosis can be associated with additional anomalies or be part of a syndrome, but more than 80% of cases are idiopathic and nonsyndromic.[3] The most commonly fused sutures in single-suture, nonsyndromic craniosynostosis are sagittal (~60%), metopic (~30%), unilateral coronal (~10%), and unilateral lambdoid (~1%).[3–5]

There are various craniofacial deformities associated with each diagnosis (**Table 1**) and there are many operative techniques for each given diagnosis and phenotype. This article will focus on open anterior cranial vault reconstruction for the diagnoses of metopic synostosis (MS) and unilateral coronal synostosis (UCS). Minimally invasive approaches (ie, strip craniectomy with post-operative helmet therapy) are covered later in this issue.

Craniofacial Center, Seattle Children's Hospital and University of Washington School of Medicine, Seattle, WA, USA
* Corresponding author. Craniofacial Center, Seattle Children's Hospital, 4800 Sand Point Way NE, Seattle, WA 98105.
E-mail address: srinivas.susarla@seattlechildrens.org

Oral Maxillofacial Surg Clin N Am 34 (2022) 367–380
https://doi.org/10.1016/j.coms.2022.01.001
1042-3699/22/© 2022 Elsevier Inc. All rights reserved.

Table 1
Craniofacial deformities associated with single suture, nonsyndromic craniosynostosis

Deformity	Sagittal	Metopic	Unilateral Coronal	Unilateral Lambdoid
Predominant Skull shape	Scaphocephaly, long and narrow boat shaped skull	Trigonocephaly	Anterior plagiocephaly, ipsilateral forehead retrusion	Posterior Plagiocephaly, trapezium shaped head from vertex view
Anterior Cranium	Frontal bossing	Triangular shaped forehead	Ipsilateral flattening of forehead contralateral frontal bossing ipsilateral deviation of nasal root contralateral deviation of nasal tip	Contralateral frontal bossing
Orbital Deformity	——	Hypotelorism, lateral orbital retrusion	Harlequin deformity: superior displacement of ipsilateral lesser wing of sphenoid, ipsilateral tail and narrow orbit, ipsilateral raised eyebrow Wide palpebral fissure	—
Middle Cranium	Decreased upper parietal width	Bitemporal narrowing	—	Ipsilateral occipitomastoid bulge
Auricular Deformity	——	——	Ipsilateral ear displaced anterior and superior	Ipsilateral displaced posterior and inferior
Posterior Cranium	Midline occipital protuberance	Compensatory occipitoparietal widening	—	Ridging on fused lambdoid suture, parallelogram-shaped head from posterior view

CLINICAL PRESENTATION

Craniosynostosis is usually diagnosed in the first few weeks of age, and often at birth. The parents or the pediatrician will note an abnormal head shape (see **Table 1**, **Fig. 1**) and will refer the child to a craniofacial surgeon or neurosurgeon. Physical examination by an experienced clinician can be diagnostic, though this can be confirmed using a low-dose CT scan which also provides information about the underlying brain.[6,7] On initial presentation, it is essential to differentiate craniosynostosis from deformational or positional plagiocephaly, as these diagnoses may be unclear to primary care providers.[8,9]

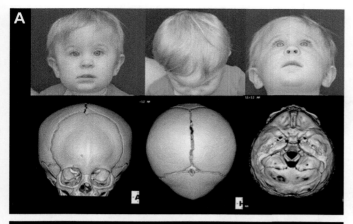
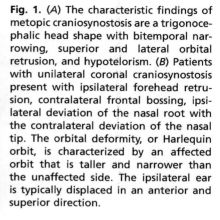

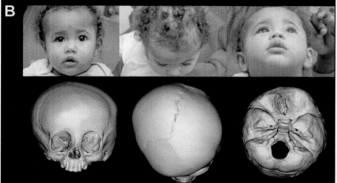

Fig. 1. (A) The characteristic findings of metopic craniosynostosis are a trigonocephalic head shape with bitemporal narrowing, superior and lateral orbital retrusion, and hypotelorism. (B) Patients with unilateral coronal craniosynostosis present with ipsilateral forehead retrusion, contralateral frontal bossing, ipsilateral deviation of the nasal root with the contralateral deviation of the nasal tip. The orbital deformity, or Harlequin orbit, is characterized by an affected orbit that is taller and narrower than the unaffected side. The ipsilateral ear is typically displaced in an anterior and superior direction.

When a diagnosis of MS or UCS is made, the family should be referred to a multi-disciplinary craniofacial center with high levels of experience.[10] Multi-disciplinary evaluation is essential, as craniosynostosis and the resultant inhibition of cranial growth results in morphologic and functional concerns, such as intracranial hypertension, visual disruption, or impaired neurologic and psychosocial development.

The risk of elevated intracranial pressure is much higher in syndromic or multi-suture synostosis. For nonsyndromic, single-suture craniosynostosis, the risk of intracranial hypertension is reported to be between 10% and 20%.[11–13] Clinical signs of elevated intracranial pressure include a tight or bulging fontanelle, failure to thrive, papilledema, "thumbprinting" or "copper-beaten" appearance on CT imaging, or

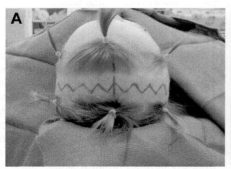
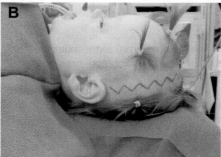

Fig. 2. (A) Standard coronal incision is shown here in this patient with right unilateral coronal synostosis. The incision is marked in a zigzag pattern to avoid forming a part along the scar. The incision is started 1.5 cm posterior and 1.5 cm superior to the helical root, with the first limb directed posteriorly (B).

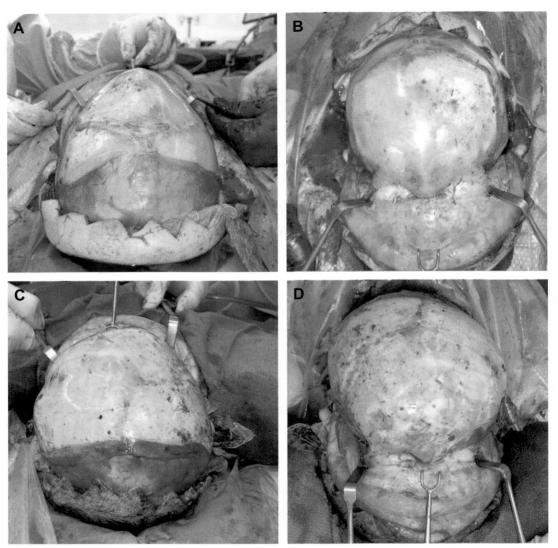

Fig. 3. Exposure for fronto-orbital advancement is shown for a patient with metopic synostosis (*A, B*) and unilateral coronal synostosis (*C, D*). The posterior extent of the exposure is just posterior to the origins of the temporalis muscles, which are reflected with the anterior scalp flap. The anterior exposure extends to the zygomatic bodies laterally and just past the nasofrontal suture in the midline. The internal orbital exposure is bounded medially by the medial canthal ligaments and laterally by the orbital floor at the inferior orbital fissure.

small ventricles with minimal extra-axial fluid on CT imaging. Elevated intracranial pressure can also result in papilledema and optic nerve atrophy, so all patients with craniosynostosis should be evaluated by an ophthalmologist. Neurocognitive development and the impact of surgery in craniosynostosis is still relatively unknown, with some data showing the operative management of craniosynostosis results in improved IQ scores when compared with unoperated patients.[14]

Both MS and UCS are managed operatively. However, the optimal timing and the type of surgical correction vary widely among craniofacial centers. Some centers recommend an endoscopic suturectomy with springs[15] or followed by postoperative helmeting,[16,17] which is typically performed in children less than 6 months of age. In patients presenting beyond this age range or in situations whereby families prefer a single-stage procedure without the need for postsurgical orthotics, open cranial vault reconstruction via fronto-orbital

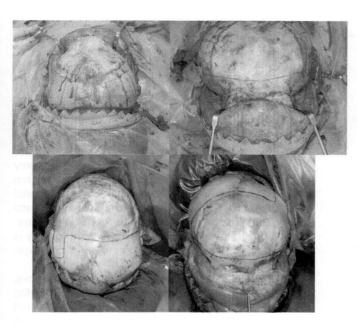

Fig. 4. Following exposure, bifrontal craniotomies and bandeau osteotomies are marked. The bifrontal craniotomy is marked posterior to the coronal suture. The bandeau osteotomy is marked 1.5 to 2.0 cm superior to the apex of the supraorbital rims in metopic synostosis and the normal supraorbital rim in UCS. In MS, barrel stave cuts are marked in the parietal bones to allow for middle vault expansion.

advancement (FOA) has long been the standard of care for anterior cranial vault deformities and remains so at our center. We typically perform FOA around 9 to 12 months of age.[18,19]

FRONTO-ORBITAL ADVANCEMENT IN METOPIC SYNOSTOSIS

The metopic suture is unique, as it is the first suture to fuse in the normal skull around 8 months, and sometimes as early as 3 months of age.[20,21] However, mild shape abnormalities that are detected in late infancy may be due to metopic ridging, not MS. It is critical to differentiate metopic ridge from MS, to avoid unnecessary diagnostics or surgery. In a large review of 282 patients with metopic ridging versus synostosis at our institution, Birgfeld and colleagues found the most common radiographic findings associated with MS.[22] Presence of 3 or more of the following findings was diagnostic for 96% of patients with MS: omega sign, interorbital narrowing, upper orbital narrowing, frontal bone tangent intersects orbital midline or medial, posteriorly displaced lateral frontal bone, straight lateral frontal bone, pulled anterior fontanelle, and upsloping lateral orbital rim.[22] There have been many attempts at clarifying diagnostic criteria for MS,[23] including morphometric analysis of CT scans to calculate the interfrontal angle[24] or even machine learning.[25]

Fronto-orbital advancement in MS aims to expand the bitemporal constriction, correct the hypoteloric orbit, and expand the triangular-shaped frontal bone to correct the deformity, frontal lobe distortion, and allow brain growth to continue normally (see **Fig. 1**A). This is achieved with a bifrontal craniotomy, rounding and reshaping of the frontal bone, and widening and rounding of the orbital bandeau. Surgery can occasionally include parietal bone grafts, intranasal bone grafts, lateral canthopexy, and the use of resorbable fixation, though none of these have been associated with changing aesthetic outcomes in MS.[26] Postoperative length of stay averages around 4 to 6 days, often with one planned night in the intensive care unit (ICU).[27,28]

The Oxford Group examined 202 patients who underwent surgery for MS and found 17.8% of patients with late temporal hollowing.[27] Similarly, a study from Washington University and Boston Children's Hospital showed a progressive decrease in frontal width postoperatively.[29] A study on 118 patients with MS from Children's Hospital of Philadelphia found that only 14.4% of had normal craniofacial aesthetics on long-term postoperative follow-up.[26] They found that though 54.2% had temporal hollowing, 47.5% had lateral orbital retrusion, 31.4% had frontal bone irregularities, and 4.2% had brow irregularities, only 6.1% had a surgical revision related to cranial abnormalities.[26] They also found that longer follow-up was independently associated with poor aesthetic outcomes, suggesting that abnormal frontal appearance may plague most patients with MS as they approach maturity.[26]

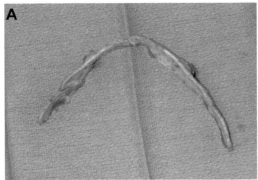

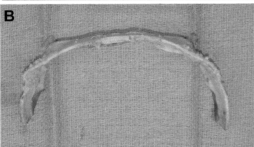

Fig. 5. Bandeau reshaping in metopic synostosis. The bandeau segment will have an angle between the supraorbital rim and tenon that approaches 180°, with an associated narrowing of the inter-orbital distance (*A*). Reshaping the bandeau requires closing wedge osteotomies placed just posterior to the fronto-zygomatic pillars, along with increasing the inter-orbital distance by using a midline calvarial bone graft (*B*). The constructed bandeau position may be stabilized with a combination of stainless-steel wires, resorbable sutures, and resorbable plates.

FRONTO-ORBITAL ADVANCEMENT IN UNILATERAL CORONAL SYNOSTOSIS

The restriction of growth perpendicular to the fused coronal suture results in an asymmetric and varied deformity that makes it one of the most challenging of the isolated synostoses to correct surgically.[30] UCS results in ipsilateral forehead flattening, contralateral frontal bossing, midfacial twist, skull base twist, and an ipsilateral Harlequin orbital deformity (see **Fig. 1**B). The Harlequin orbital deformity is the result of the superior displacement of the ipsilateral lesser wing of the sphenoid, causing the ipsilateral orbital to be both taller and narrower than the contralateral side.[18] The midfacial twist results in an ipsilateral deviation of the nasal root and contralateral deviation of the nasal tip. The skull base twists toward the fused coronal suture, resulting in an ipsilaterally deviated chin, and an anteriorly and superiorly displaced ipsilateral ear.

Fronto-orbital advancement for UCS aims to correct the cranial and orbital components of the deformity but does not directly affect the midface or skull base. Due to the ipsilateral forehead flattening with the contralateral protrusion, the frontal bone and orbital bandeau are reshaped such that the ipsilateral orbital rim is brought forward while the contralateral orbital rim is retruded.[18,31] The ipsilateral orbital rim is also brought inferiorly, to correct the Harlequin orbital deformity, but this does not widen the ipsilateral orbit.[18] Surgery can also include ipsilateral superior orbital rim onlay bone grafts,[31] contralateral interpositional orbital bone grafts,[32] shortening of the ipsilateral lateral orbital rim,[18] or be isolated to a hemi-orbital bandeau.[33] Postoperative length of stay is similar to that in MS, ranging around 4 to 6 days, often with one night in the ICU.[28,32]

The Children's Hospital of Philadelphia group reported on the aesthetic outcomes following FOA for 176 patients with UCS and found that only 10.2% had normal craniofacial aesthetics on long-term follow-up.[32] They found that 75% of patients had supraorbital retrusion, 55.1% of patients had temporal hollowing, and 4.0% had occipital abnormalities.[32] Surgical revisions were required in 22.7% of patients, most of which were only cranial bone grafting or alloplastic cranioplasty.[32] They found that severity of the deformity gave a five times increased risk of developing temporal hollowing, though the overcorrection of the bandeau resulted in three times decreased risk of temporal hollowing.[32] The group at Seattle Children's Hospital performed a comprehensive, 3-

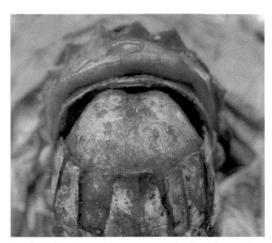

Fig. 6. Following placement of the bandeau, there will be a notable expansion in the anterior cranial base, with a rounded supraorbital framework. Note the outfractured parietal barrel staves, creating a middle vault expansion.

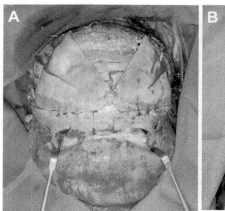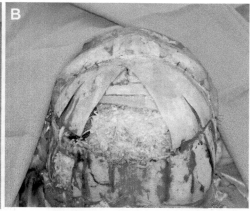

Fig. 7. Frontal cranioplasty is accomplished using multiple radial osteotomies within the bone flap and contouring the flap margins to align with the bandeau framework. The frontal bone flap is secured to the bandeau using resorbable sutures (*A*). Middle vault expansion is accomplished using multiple barrel stave osteotomies within the parietal bones. Following the advancement of the forehead, there will be an interpositional gap between the frontal bone flap and native parietal bones. This gap is grafted with cortical and particulate calvarial bone autograft (*B*).

dimensional morphometric study on 43 patients with UCS compared with controls found that patients who had an overcorrection of the bandeau were five times more likely to have a symmetric result at long-term follow-up.[18] They also found that patients with more severe brow retrusion were four times more likely to have persistent asymmetry at follow-up.[18] Shortening of the ipsilateral rim resulted in the normalization of the orbital height ratio, but there was no change in the orbital width ratio, with the ipsilateral orbit narrower at all time points studied.[18] Midfacial twist improved over time but did not normalize, and the skull base twist did not change significantly postoperatively.[18] Thus, there is ample room for the improvement of the surgical management of UCS, at the skull base, midface, and cranial vault levels.

Due to the significant orbital deformity and surgical instrumentation of the area, there are often associated ocular findings such as strabismus, aniso-astigmatism, and amblyopia.[34,35] A systematic review by Dencarelli and colleagues found these rates to be as high as 19% to 100%, 15% to 92%, and 3% to 56%, respectively.[35] Many surgeons have looked for ways to reduce the risk of developing these findings postoperatively. The Boston Children's Hospital group reported that patients treated with endoscopic strip craniectomy were less likely to develop all 3 of these findings or require corrective ophthalmologic surgery when compared with infants treated with traditional FOA.[34,36] Particularly regarding strabismus, Hoppe and Taylor found that patients undergoing frontal orbital distraction osteogenesis versus FOA developed less strabismus postoperatively.

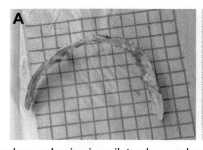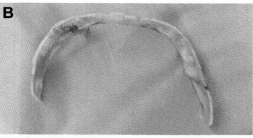

Fig. 8. Bandeau reshaping in unilateral coronal synostosis. The bandeau segment will have an excessively obtuse angle between the supraorbital rim and tenon extension with associated retrusion of the supraorbital rim on the affected side (*A*). Reshaping the bandeau requires a closing wedge osteotomy placed just posterior to the fronto-zygomatic pillar, along with a midline osteotomy to allow the bandeau to be "untwisted" – bringing the affected supraorbital rim forward and down (*B*). The constructed bandeau position may be stabilized with a combination of stainless-steel wires, resorbable sutures, and resorbable plates.

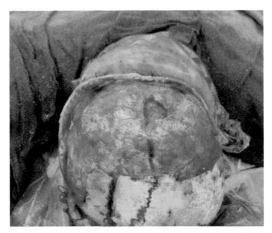

Fig. 9. Following the placement of the bandeau, there will be a notable expansion in the anterior cranial base on the affected side, with the overcorrection of the supraorbital rim on the affected side relative to the unaffected side.

These findings, however, are tempered by the fact that infants who underwent endoscopic or distraction osteogenesis techniques were found to be significantly younger at the time of operation when compared with those who underwent open FOA. This may suggest that earlier intervention portends improved outcomes rather than any particular technique.[37] However, as minimally invasive options can generally be offered at a younger age than FOA, this remains a potential advantage of these approaches over FOA.

Fronto-Orbital Advancement – Operative Technique

We use a coronal incision for access to the orbits and anterior cranial vault. The incision is marked in a zigzag fashion, starting 1.5 cm superior and posterior to the helical origin, with the first limb directed posteriorly (**Fig. 2**). The posterior scalp flap is elevated first in the subgaleal plane to a point just posterior to the origins of the temporalis muscles. A pericranial incision is then made here and the temporalis muscles are elevated contiguous with the anterior scalp flap to the level of the superior orbital rims. The fronto-zygomatic pillar is then exposed down to its junction with the zygomatic body. A 2/3 internal orbital dissection is then completed, extending from just above the medial canthal ligaments medially to the inferior orbital fissure laterally. This exposure affords access to the orbits and frontal and parietal bones (**Fig. 3**).

After the exposure, the lateral orbital osteotomies are completed, starting at or slightly above the junction of the fronto-zygomatic pillar with the zygomatic body and moving posteriorly into the inferior orbital fissure. The vertical osteotomy along the lateral orbital wall is then made from the inferior orbital fissure to just shy of the temporal bulge in the superolateral orbit.

Once the orbital cuts are completed on both sides, a bifrontal craniotomy is marked posterior to the coronal sutures (**Fig. 4**). In MS, additional barrel stave cuts are marked in the parietal bones to allow for middle vault expansion. Burr holes, epidural dissection, and bifrontal craniotomies are performed in conjunction with the neurosurgical team. The frontal bone flap is removed and the dura is carefully inspected for injury. Any dural rents or tears are repaired using - 4-0 Nurolon suture.

The bandeau osteotomies are then completed, beginning with the tenon extensions bilaterally,

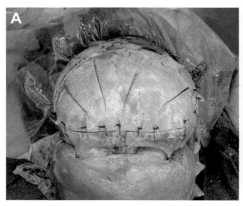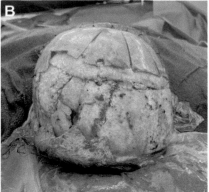

Fig. 10. Frontal cranioplasty is accomplished using multiple radial osteotomies within the bone flap and contouring the flap margins to align with the bandeau framework. The frontal bone flap is secured to the bandeau using resorbable sutures (*A*). Following the advancement of the forehead, there will be an interpositional gap between the frontal bone flap and native parietal bone, greater on the affected side. This gap is grafted with particulate calvarial bone autograft (*B*).

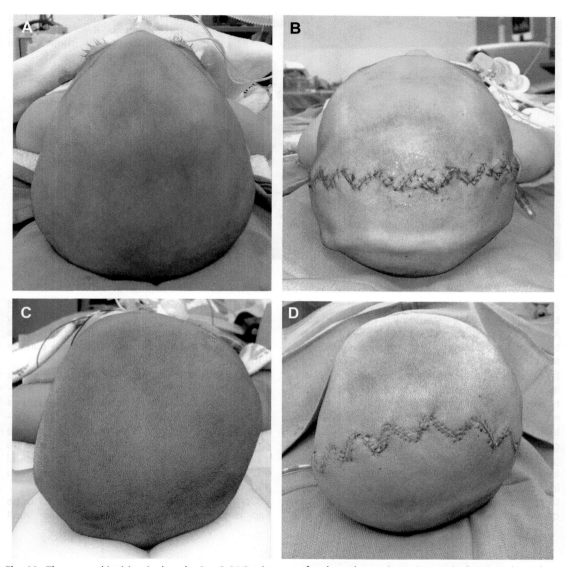

Fig. 11. The coronal incision is closed using 3-0 Vicryl sutures for the galea and running and interrupted 4-0 chromic gut sutures for the scalp (*A, B*: metopic synostosis; *C, D*: right unilateral coronal synostosis). Galeal scoring at the time of initial anterior and posterior scalp flap elevation affords an opportunity for intraoperative expansion of the scalp soft tissue, easily permitting a tension-free closure following skeletal reconstruction.

which are stopped just shy of the fronto-zygomatic suture. Next, the midline bandeau osteotomy is completed just above the cribriform plate. The midline osteotomy is then connected to orbital roof cuts bilaterally, which are then transitioned to connect with the vertical limbs of the lateral orbital wall cuts, at which point the saw blade will leave the orbit and progress through the sphenoid wing, terminating extra-cranially to connect with the craniotomy cut for the tenon extensions. The bandeau is then liberated, and the globes

are inspected for evidence of periorbital tears or adnexal injury. Periorbital tears are generally not consequential, but may result in increased or prolonged periorbital swelling postoperatively.

Bandeau Reshaping and Frontal Cranioplasty – Metopic Synostosis

The bandeau in metopic craniosynostosis is narrow and angulated (**Fig. 5**A). Reshaping is directed toward increasing the interorbital width

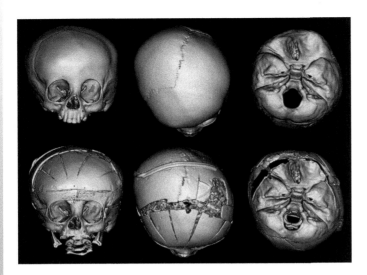

Fig. 12. Pre- (top row) and post (bottom row) three-dimensional images show the immediate changes in cranio-orbital morphology in this patient with left unilateral coronal craniosynostosis.

(exocanthion–exocanthion distance) and interfrontal angles. A midline osteotomy is performed first, followed by closing wedge osteotomies just posterior to the fronto-zygomatic pillars. Greenstick fractures are then created at the junction of the tenon extension with the frontozygomatic pillars, and an angle of approximately 135° is created between the tenon extension and the supraorbital rim. Each individual hemi-bandeau segment is then replaced to be evaluated in situ. The resulting gap at the midline is measured and a cortical bone graft is harvested from the parietal region to allow for transverse expansion of the bandeau, increasing the exocanthion–exocanthion distance to approximately 90 mm (some overcorrection is desirable, in the recognition of the transverse relapse noted over the long term as described above). The constructed bandeau is stabilized by using resorbable plates on the endocranial surface and wires or sutures on the ectocranial surface (**Fig. 5**B).

The constructed bandeau is then inset into a slightly advanced position and secured using 26-gauge stainless-steel wires or resorbable sutures at the nasofrontal junction in the midline and zygomatic bodies laterally. Resorbable plates are placed at the tenon extensions. There should be a notable expansion in the bitemporal and lateral orbital regions following the inset of the bandeau (**Fig. 6**).

Once the bandeau is affixed, the frontal bone flap is contoured to afford an anterior vault

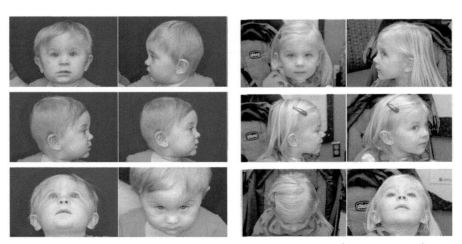

Fig. 13. Preoperative (*left*) and 2-year postoperative images (*right*) are shown for a patient with metopic craniosynostosis who was treated with fronto-orbital advancement at 12 months of age.

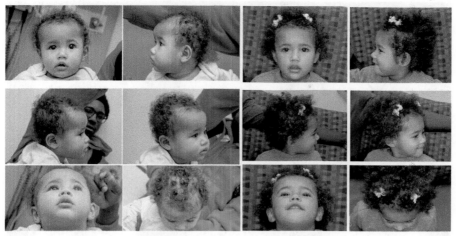

Fig. 14. Preoperative (*left*) and 2-year postoperative images (*right*) are shown for a patient with left unilateral coronal synostosis who was treated with fronto-orbital advancement at 12 months of age.

expansion and parietal barrel staves are created to afford a middle vault expansion. Radial osteotomies in the bone flap are performed to allow expansion. When the significant expansion is needed splitting the bone flap in the midline is sometimes required. Bony gaps created by the expansion of the frontal bone flap and parietal barrel staves are then filled with calvarial autograft, including morcellated particulate calvarial graft mixed with fibrin sealant, which is harvested from the endocortex of the frontal bone flap. The expanded bone flap is then secured in place using resorbable sutures (**Fig. 7**).

Bandeau Reshaping and Frontal Cranioplasty – Unicoronal Synostosis

The bandeau in unicoronal craniosynostosis is asymmetric related to the orbital deformity. Reshaping is directed toward increasing the orbital width, decreasing the orbital height, and narrowing the angle between the supraorbital rim and tenon extension on the affected side (**Fig. 8**A). A midline osteotomy is performed first, followed by a closing wedge osteotomy just posterior to the fronto-zygomatic pillar on the affected side. Greenstick fractures are then created at the midline and frontozygomatic pillar, and an angle

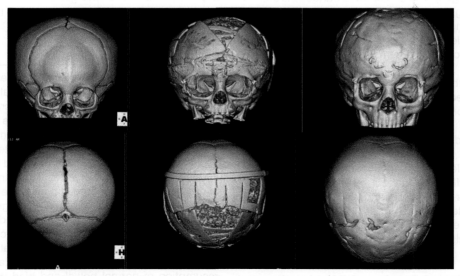

Fig. 15. Three-dimensional CT evaluation demonstrating improved cranio-orbital morphology in a patient with metopic craniosynostosis. Preoperative (*left*), immediate postoperative (*middle*), and 2-years postoperative (*right*) images are shown.

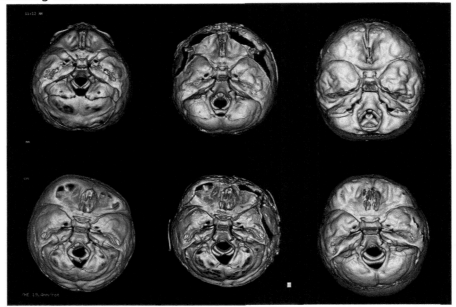

Fig. 16. Anterior skull base morphologies are shown for patients with metopic (*top row*) and right unilateral coronal (*bottom row*) synostoses preoperatively (*left images*), immediately postoperatively (*middle images*), and at 2-years postoperatively (*right images*).

of approximately 135° is created between the tenon extension and the supraorbital rim. The bandeau is then tried in, with the tenon segment on the affected side advanced and superiorly rotated, ensuring bone to bone contact with the parietal bone on that side. The final bandeau position should have the supraorbital rim on the affected side over-corrected by approximately 20% relative to the unaffected supraorbital rim (**Fig. 8**B). Significant expansion of the anterior cranial base should be apparent when viewed from above (**Fig. 9**). The constructed bandeau is affixed to the zygomatic bodies and the nasofrontal junction using 26-gauge stainless-steel wires or resorbable sutures. The tenon extensions are affixed to the parietal bone using resorbable plates.

Once the bandeau is affixed, the frontal bone flap is recontoured. Multiple radial osteotomies are performed to expand the frontal bone flap, with the affected side advanced and laterally expanded relative to the unaffected side. The frontal bone flap is affixed to the bandeau using resorbable sutures. Advancement of the forehead on the affected side will result in a sizable full-thickness calvarial defect, which is grafted using particulate calvarial graft (harvested from the endocortex of the frontal bone flap) mixed with fibrin sealant (**Fig. 10**).

Closure

The anterior and posterior scalp flaps are then readvanced over the reconstructed fronto-orbital framework. Galeal scoring of the flaps is best undertaken immediately after they are elevated, which affords time for intra-operative soft-tissue expansion while the bony work is completed. A subgaleal drain is placed in the posterior aspect of the wound bed (to allow for dependent drainage) and brought out behind the ear, with the drain site being at the junction of the hair-bearing and non–hair-bearing postauricular skin, which allows for easy removal and an inconspicuous scar. The scalp is then closed in layers using 3-0 Vicryl sutures for the galea and running and interrupted 4-0 chromic gut sutures for the scalp skin (**Fig. 11**).

Postoperative Care

Our postoperative care protocol includes an immediate postoperative CT scan to evaluate the reconstruction and assess for any intracranial abnormalities (**Fig. 12**). Concerning findings necessitating intervention or further management are quite rare (0.55%).[6] Patients are admitted to the ICU for the first night after surgery, and then the surgical floor for care thereafter. The skin incision is dressed with antibiotic ointment twice daily for the first week postoperatively. Discharge criteria are pain controlled with oral medications, nausea/emesis that is minimal or controlled with oral medications, resolution of periorbital swelling such that at least one eye opens spontaneously, resumption of normal bowel and bladder habits, and adequate oral intake. Patients are seen at 2 to 4-weeks postoperatively, and then annually to assess for healing (**Figs. 13** and **14**). At 2-years postoperatively, CT imaging is repeated to assess for bony healing (**Figs. 15** and **16**). Any critical-sized bone defects (≥ 3 cm^2) are followed until age 5 to 6, at which time secondary cranioplasty is considered for persistent defects.

CLINICS CARE POINTS

- Fronto-orbital advancement remains a valuable tool for the treatment of the cranio-orbital deficiency seen in metopic and unilateral craniosynostoses.
- The structural components of the fronto-orbital advancement are the frontal bone flap and orbital bandeau segment.
- In metopic craniosynostosis, the bandeau will need to be widened in the midline and the angles between the tenon and supraorbital rim segments narrowed. The frontal cranioplasty serves to widen the forehead, with interpositional gaps typically found in the midline and between the frontal and parietal bones. Overcorrection of the transverse expansion is indicated, due to the known relapse in this dimension.[29]
- In unilateral coronal craniosynostosis, the bandeau will need to be "untwisted" by advancing the supraorbital rim anteriorly, narrowing the angle between the tenon segment and supraorbital rim, as well as decreasing the height and expanding the width of the orbit on the affected side. The frontal cranioplasty serves to widen and advance the forehead on the affected side, with interpositional gaps typically found between the frontal and parietal bones on the affected side. The orbital rim on the affected side should be overcorrected by at least 20% in the sagittal dimension, due to the well-recognized potential for relapse.[18]

REFERENCES

1. Virchow H. Ueber drn Cretinismus, namentlich in Franken, und ueber pathologishe Schaedelforamen. Verh Phys Med Ges Wuerzbg 1851;2:230–71.
2. Persing JA, Jane JA, Shaffrey M. Virchow and the pathogenesis of craniosynostosis: a translation of his original work. Plast Reconstr Surg 1989;83(4):738–42.
3. Di Rocco F, Arnaud E, Renier D. Evolution in the frequency of nonsyndromic craniosynostosis: Clinical article. J Neurosurg Pediatr 2009;4(1):21–5.
4. Cornelissen M, Ottelander B den, Rizopoulos D, et al. Increase of prevalence of craniosynostosis. J Cranio-Maxillofacial Surg 2016;44(9):1273–9.
5. Selber J, Reid RR, Chike-Obi CJ, et al. The changing epidemiologic spectrum of single-suture synostoses. Plast Reconstr Surg 2008;122(2):527–33.
6. Ahammout C, Perez FA, Birgfeld CB, et al. Evaluating the utility of routine computed tomography scans after cranial vault reconstruction for children with craniosynostosis. Plast Reconstr Surg 2021;148(1):63e–70e.
7. Morton RP, Reynolds RM, Ramakrishna R, et al. Low-dose head computed tomography in children: a single institutional experience in pediatric radiation risk reduction. J Neurosurg Pediatr 2013;12(4):406–10.
8. Huang MHS, Mouradian WE, Cohen SR, et al. The differential diagnosis of abnormal head shapes: Separating craniosynostosis from positional deformities and normal variants. Cleft Palate J 1998;35(3):204–11.
9. Birgfeld CB, Heike C. Distinguishing between lambdoid craniosynostosis and deformational plagiocephaly: a review of this paradigm shift in clinical decision-making and lesson for the future. Craniomaxillofac Trauma Reconstr 2020;13(4):248–52.
10. Wes AM, Mazzaferro D, Naran S, et al. Craniosynostosis surgery: Does hospital case volume impact outcomes or cost? Plast Reconstr Surg 2017;140(5):711e–8e.
11. Tamburrini G, Caldarelli M, Massimi L, et al. Intracranial pressure monitoring in children with single suture and complex craniosynostosis: a review. Child's Nerv Syst 2005;21(10):913–21.
12. Hayward R. Venous hypertension and craniosynostosis. Child's Nerv Syst 2005;21(10):880–8.
13. Gault DT, Renier D, Marchac D, et al. Intracranial pressure and intracranial volume in children with craniosynostosis. Plast Reconstr Surg 1992;90(3):377–81.
14. Speltz ML, Collett BR, Wallace ER, et al. Intellectual and academic functioning of school-age children with single-suture craniosynostosis. Pediatrics 2015;135(3):e615–23.
15. Lauritzen CGK, Davis C, Ivarsson A, et al. The evolving role of springs in craniofacial surgery: the first 100 clinical cases. Plast Reconstr Surg 2008;121:545–54.
16. Riordan CP, Zurakowski D, Meier PM, et al. Minimally Invasive Endoscopic Surgery for Infantile Craniosynostosis: A Longitudinal Cohort Study. J Pediatr 2020;216:142–9.e2.
17. Pressler MP, Hallac RR, Geisler EL, et al. Comparison of head shape outcomes in metopic synostosis using limited strip craniectomy and open vault reconstruction techniques. Cleft Palate Craniofac J 2021;58(6):669–77.
18. Liu MT, Khechoyan DY, Susarla SM, et al. Evolution of bandeau shape, orbital morphology, and

craniofacial twist after fronto-orbital advancement for isolated unilateral coronal synostosis: a case-control Study of 2-Year Outcomes. Plast Reconstr Surg 2019;143(6):1703–11.

19. Birgfeld CB, Dufton L, Naumann H, et al. Safety of open cranial vault surgery for single-suture craniosynostosis: a case for the multidisciplinary team. J Craniofac Surg 2015;26(7):2052–8.

20. Vu HL, Panchal J, Parker EE, et al. The timing of physiologic closure of the metopic suture: A review of 159 patients using reconstructed 3D CT scans of the craniofacial region. J Craniofac Surg 2001; 12(6):527–32.

21. Weinzweig J, Kirschner RE, Farley A, et al. Metopic synostosis: defining the temporal sequence of normal suture fusion and differentiating it from synostosis on the basis of computed tomography images. Plast Reconstr Surg 2003;112(5):1211–8.

22. Birgfeld CB, Saltzman BS, Hing AV, et al. Making the diagnosis: metopic ridge versus metopic craniosynostosis. J Craniofac Surg 2013;24(1):178–85.

23. Nassar AH, Mercan E, Massenburg BB, et al. What craniometric measure best defines metopic synostosis? Plast Reconstr Surg - Glob Open 2019;7(8S-2): 201–2.

24. Wood BC, Mendoza CS, Oh AK, et al. What's in a name? Accurately diagnosing metopic craniosynostosis using a computational approach. Plast Reconstr Surg 2016;137(1):205–13.

25. Bhalodia R, Dvoracek LA, Ayyash AM, et al. Quantifying the severity of metopic craniosynostosis: a pilot study application of machine learning in craniofacial surgery. J Craniofac Surg 2020;31(3): 697–701.

26. Wes AM, Paliga JT, Goldstein JA, et al. An evaluation of complications, revisions, and long-term aesthetic outcomes in nonsyndromic metopic craniosynostosis. Plast Reconstr Surg 2014;133(6):1453–64.

27. Natghian H, Song M, Jayamohan J, et al. Long-term results in isolated metopic synostosis: The Oxford experience over 22 years. Plast Reconstr Surg 2018;142(4):509E–15E.

28. Massenburg BB, Nassar AH, Hopper RA. National database reported outcomes following craniosynostosis reconstruction. J Craniofac Surg 2020;31(1):154–7.

29. Patel KB, Skolnick GB, Mulliken JB. Anthropometric outcomes following fronto-orbital advancement for metopic synostosis. Plast Reconstr Surg 2016; 137(5):1539–47.

30. McCarthy JG, Glasberg SB, Cutting CB, et al. Twenty-year experience with early surgery for craniosynostosis: I. Isolated craniofacial synostosis–results and unsolved problems. Plast Reconstr Surg 1995;96(2):272–83.

31. Grant JH, Roberts TS, Loeser JD, et al. Onlay bone graft augmentation for refined correction of coronal synostosis. Cleft Palate Craniofac J 2002;39(5): 546–54.

32. Taylor JA, Paliga JT, Wes AM, et al. A critical evaluation of long-term aesthetic outcomes of fronto-orbital advancement and cranial vault remodeling in nonsyndromic unicoronal craniosynostosis. Plast Reconstr Surg 2015;135(1):220–31.

33. Seal SKF, Steinbok P, Courtemanche DJ. The cranial orbital buttress technique for nonsyndromic unicoronal and metopic craniosynostosis. Neurosurg Focus 2015;38(5):1–10.

34. Elhusseiny AM, MacKinnon S, Zurakowski D, et al. Long-term ophthalmic outcomes in 120 children with unilateral coronal synostosis: a 20-year retrospective analysis. J Am Assoc Pediatr Ophthalmol Strabismus 2021;25(2):76.e1–5.

35. Gencarelli JR, Murphy A, Samargandi OA, et al. Ophthalmologic outcomes following fronto-orbital advancement for unicoronal craniosynostosis. J Craniofac Surg 2016;27(7):1629–35.

36. Isaac KV, Mackinnon S, Dagi LR, et al. Nonsyndromic unilateral coronal synostosis: a comparison of fronto-orbital advancement and endoscopic suturectomy. Plast Reconstr Surg 2019;143(3):838–48.

37. Hoppe IC, Taylor JA. A Cohort Study of strabismus rates following correction of the unicoronal craniosynostosis deformity: conventional bilateral fronto-orbital advancement versus fronto-orbital distraction osteogenesis. J Craniofac Surg 2021;32(7):2362–5.

Management of Unicoronal and Metopic Synostoses
Minimally Invasive Approaches

Gabriel M. Hayek, DMD, MD[a], David F. Jimenez, MD[b],
David M. Yates, DMD, MD[c],*

KEYWORDS

- Craniosynostosis • Metopic • Trigonocephaly • Coronal • Unicoronal • Endoscopic
- Minimally invasive

KEY POINTS

- Early endoscopic-assisted surgery is associated with decreased blood loss, operating time, transfusion rates, hospital stay and costs, pain, and swelling when compared with open procedures.
- Endoscopic-assisted repair appears to correct downstream facial deformities.
- There are less reoperative cases necessary with endoscopic-assisted repair.

INTRODUCTION

Unicoronal synostosis has an incidence of approximately 0.4:1000 births and is the third most common single-suture synostosis[1] (**Fig. 1**). Although most cases are sporadic, there is a familial incidence of up to 8% of single-suture cases. The clinical presentation includes orbital misalignment with vertical dystopia, proptosis, ipsilateral frontal plagiocephaly with compensatory overgrowth of the contralateral frontal bone, cranial scoliosis, and contralateral nasal tip deviation. The classic "harlequin" sign presents as ipsilateral elevation and lateral retraction of the orbit. Many consider this to be the most disfiguring of the single-suture synostoses, as there will be downstream effects on the facial skeleton owing to twisting of the craniomaxillofacial complex (**Fig. 2**). Failure to correct the deformity early can result in significant and permanent ophthalmologic sequelae, including amblyopia or loss of vision in the eye.[1,2]

Metopic synostosis has traditionally had an incidence of 1:15,000 live births, although it is becoming more common and approaching 1:5000 live births[3,4] (**Fig. 3**). It is now the second most commonly affected single-suture synostosis after the sagittal suture.[5,6] The metopic suture is unique because it is normal to be closed as early as 3 months, raising concerns that the increased reported incidence is due to overdiagnosis.[7,8] It is the only major cranial suture permitted to fuse before adulthood.[9] Metopic synostosis results from early closure of the metopic suture, resulting in lateral growth restriction of the frontal bones and bitemporal narrowing, causing a triangular-shaped forehead known as trigonocephaly.[3,5,10–13] A midline anterior calvarial ridge on the forehead is also present over the stenosed suture.[14] Hypotelorism results from deficient lateral movement of the orbits. There are few to no findings in the mid and lower face[9] (**Fig. 4**). Additional findings that can aid in the diagnosis of metopic synostosis

---

[a] Division of Oral and Maxillofacial Surgery, Department of Craniofacial Sciences, University of Connecticut, Farmington, CT, USA; [b] Pediatric Neurosurgery, El Paso Children's Hospital, El Paso, TX 79905, USA; [c] Division of Cleft and Craniofacial Surgery, Department of Oral and Maxillofacial Surgery, El Paso Children's Hospital, El Paso, TX 79905, USA
* Corresponding author. El Paso Children's Hospital, 5340 El Paso Drive, Suite M, El Paso, TX 79905.
E-mail address: yates@hdofs.com

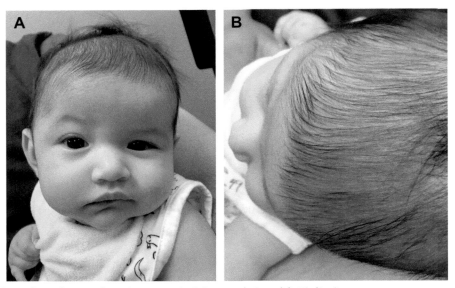

Fig. 1. Right unilateral coronal craniosynostosis. (*A*) Frontal view. (*B*). Bird's view.

include epicanthal folds, biparietal widening, and raised brows. If a diagnosis of metopic synostosis versus metopic ridge remains in question, a computed tomographic (CT) scan may help evaluate for supportive findings of metopic synostosis, including a metopic notch or a significant interfrontal angle.[15]

Today, cranial and facial deformational changes related to craniosynostosis remain challenging to treat, and surgeons continue to debate the merits of open calvarial remodeling versus endoscopic-assisted techniques.[1,16–34] Anterior calvarial synostoses, including the metopic and coronal sutures, are particularly challenging, as the relation to the facial skeleton can result in marked and severe cranial and facial deformities. Proponents of early surgery argue that the brain quadruples in size in the first year of life, allowing appropriate advancement of the frontal bone and supraorbital rims in an organically natural way, similar to normal cranial development.

Those who advocate for delayed open surgery argue that waiting for craniofacial growth relies less on brain development and that patients are better able to tolerate potential blood loss. In addition, they argue that immediate and complete correction of the deformity may be achieved at the time of an open repair. The literature is replete with techniques for open surgery, resulting in data that show that open calvarial remodeling is inconsistent in treatment outcomes and associated with numerous postoperative problems and complications.[35–37] Open surgery is associated with increased blood transfusion rates and longer hospital stays. Open corrections are also prone to

regression and visible postsurgical deformities, which generally are not fully present until about 4 years postoperatively.[38] Furthermore, delayed open correction does not significantly improve complex orbital deformities or the maxillary, mandibular, and nasal deformities, which frequently occur in unicoronal synostosis and which will persist and worsen into adulthood.[39,40]

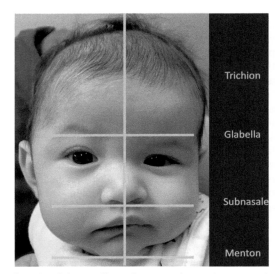

Fig. 2. Right unilateral coronal craniosynostosis; twisting of the craniomaxillofacial complex. Note vertical dystopia, poorly projected affected side superior orbital rim, superior portion of nasal bone deviated to the affected side with nasal tip deviation toward unaffected side, chin deviation toward unaffected side, and right-sided frontal flattening.

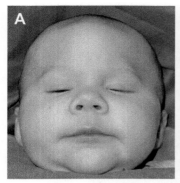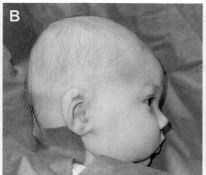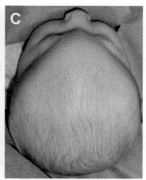

Fig. 3. Metopic craniosynostosis. (*A*) Frontal view. (*B*) Right profile view. (*C*) Bird's view.

The development of minimally invasive techniques has made the procedure safer while providing excellent deformity correction at a lower cost.[41]

UNICORONAL SYNOSTOSIS

The patient is placed supine on a horseshoe headrest, with the head slightly rotated to the contralateral side. After induction of general anesthesia, a baseline hemoglobin and hematocrit are obtained using just a few cubic centimeters of blood via a heel stick.[1,2,42] No arterial line, central venous line, or Foley catheter is needed, given the procedure's minimally invasive nature. Two peripheral intravenous lines are placed, and a precordial Doppler is used to monitor for venous air embolism. A heating unit (Bair Hugger) prevents hypothermia. A single dose of prophylactic antibiotics, as well as a 50-mg/kg dose of tranexamic acid, is administered immediately before surgery. The patient is sterilely prepared with a povidone-iodine solution and draped. Corneal protectors with an ophthalmic lubricant are used to prevent corneal abrasion.

A 2-cm incision is made over the stephanion (junction of the coronal suture with the superior temporal line), halfway between the anterior fontanelle and the pterion (H-shaped junction of the greater wing of the sphenoid bone, squamous portion of the temporal bone, frontal bone, and parietal bone) on the side of the affected suture. It is noted that the proposed osteotomy is actually posterior to the fused suture and carried inferiorly to the squamosal suture (**Fig. 5**). This results in an easier dissection and craniectomy while achieving the same outcome of total release. Monopolar electrocautery with an extralong needle tip set at 10-W Cut and 15-W Coag is used to incise the dermis and galea. Dissection then proceeds in the subgaleal plane, between the galea and the pericranium, with the aid of a rhinoplasty lighted retractor and a 0° rigid endoscope.

The dissection is first done in a medial direction toward the anterior fontanelle, followed by the lateral direction to reach the extent of the pterion on the affected side (**Fig. 6**). The inferior portion of the lateral dissection is performed with a ribbon retractor in the subgaleal plane (**Fig. 7**).

A pediatric craniotome is then used to create a 7-mm burr hole at the incision site to access the epidural space. The burr hole is enlarged longitudinally along the suture axis for approximately 1 cm in either direction using a 4-mm Kerrison rongeur. Enlarging the burr hole allows the placement of a 30° rigid endoscope under the stenosed suture to develop the epidural space plane of dissection. The dissection is advanced in the epidural space using small, guarded suction, and the endoscope is advanced to the anterior fontanelle. Once freed from the scalp and dura, a Mayo scissors, a pituitary rongeur, or a straight Leksell rongeur is used to cut a 4- to 5-mm strip of bone up to the edge

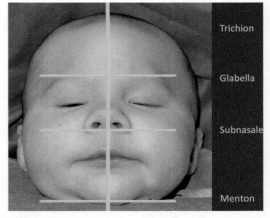

Fig. 4. Metopic craniosynostosis: facial analysis. Note hypotelorism and poorly projected lateral superior orbital rims, otherwise appropriate facial symmetry and proportions.

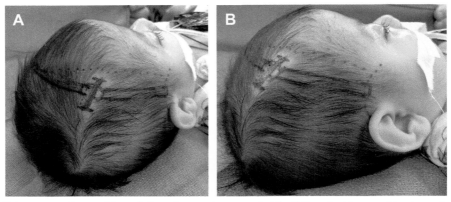

Fig. 5. (*A, B*) Intraoperative markings right unicoronal synostosis. The 2.5-cm incision marking is made at the Stephanion; the dotted line represents the synostosed right coronal suture, and inferiorly the dotted line is the open squamosal suture. The 2 solid lines represent the site of the proposed craniectomy, which is placed posterior to the proposed synostosed suture and is taken all the way to the squamosal suture.

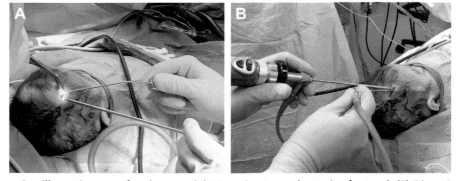

Fig. 6. Dissection illustrating use of endoscope. (*A*) Dissection toward anterior fontanel. (*B*) Dissection to squamosal suture.

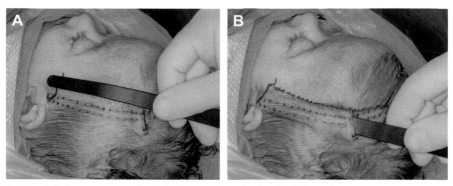

Fig. 7. (*A, B*) Use of ribbon retractor for inferior portion of subgaleal dissection.

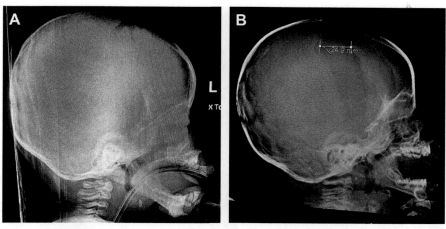

Fig. 8. Unicoronal synostosis: immediate postoperative and 3.5-months postoperative plain films demonstrating fronto-orbital advancement. (*A*) Immediate postoperative image showing 4- to 5-mm craniectomy. (*B*) 3.5-months postoperative image demonstrating 20 mm advancement as measured as site of craniectomy.

of the fontanelle, making sure the frontal bone is fully released. The endoscope is then redirected laterally toward the pterion to the open squamosal suture. Again, a 4- to 5-mm osteotomy is made, ensuring that it extends down to the squamosal suture. If inadequately released, the frontal-orbital-facial complex will fail to appropriately move forward and inferiorly.

After ensuring the separation of the entire frontal-orbital complex, osseous hemostasis is achieved using a suction-cautery unit. Often, multiple passes are required for complete hemostasis and can be performed until the bone is charred. Additional hemostasis is achieved using Surgiflo and liquid thrombin. Close inspection of the dura

and bone is performed to look for dural tears or residual bleeding. The galeal layer is closed with 4-0 Monocryl suture, and the skin is closed with Mastisol and Steri-Strips.

It should be noted that the dura overlying the coronal suture ossifies at a slower rate than over the vertex. Anterior growth of the brain also moves the frontal bone forward as much as 2 to 2.5 cm as can be seen on plain skull films postoperatively (**Fig. 8**). A large strip craniectomy can thus lead to large areas devoid of bone, and the osteotomy width should be limited to the width of the Kerrison rongeur. Following a successful surgery, compliance with helmet therapy and patience are keys to excellent results. Many times complete

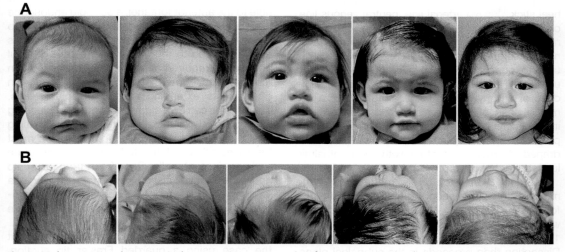

Fig. 9. Right unicoronal synostosis demonstrating progression from preoperative photograph to 24 months postoperatively. (*A*) Preoperative bird's view, 3 months, 6 months, 12 months, and 24 months postoperatively. (*B*) Preoperative bird's view, 3 months, 6 months, 12 months, and 24 months postoperatively.

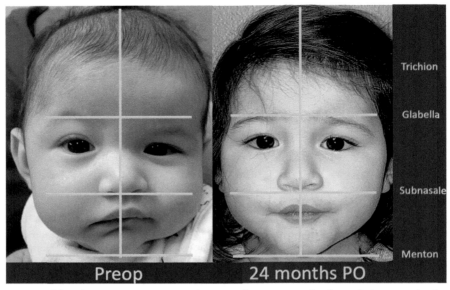

Trichion

Glabella

Subnasale

Menton

Preop   24 months PO

Fig. 10. Correction of facial twist. Preoperative and 24 months postoperative frontal photographs demonstrating significant improvement in facial asymmetry. Face is subdivided into facial thirds; significant improvement is noted in nasal deviation, mandibular deviation, orbital asymmetry, vertical dystopia, maxillary and frontal bone asymmetry. PO, postoperative; preop, preoperative.

resolution of the deformity is not appreciated until 2 to 4 years after the surgery; this is to be expected and is communicated to the parents preoperatively (**Fig. 9** and**10**).

METOPIC SYNOSTOSIS

The patient is placed supine on a horseshoe headrest. After induction of general anesthesia, a baseline hemoglobin and hematocrit are obtained using just a few cubic centimeters of blood via a heel stick.[14,42] No arterial line, central venous line, or Foley catheter is needed, given the procedure's minimally invasive nature. Two peripheral intravenous lines are placed, and a precordial Doppler is used to monitor for venous air embolism. A heating unit (Bair Hugger) prevents hypothermia. A single dose of prophylactic antibiotics, as well as a 50-mg/kg dose of tranexamic acid, is administered immediately before surgery. The patient is sterilely prepared with a povidone-iodine solution and draped. Corneal protectors with an ophthalmic lubricant are used to prevent corneal abrasion.

A 2- to 3-cm incision is made across the metopic suture between the hairline and anterior fontanelle (**Fig. 11**). Monopolar electrocautery with an extralong needle tip set at 10-W Cut and 15-W Coag is used to incise the dermis and galea. Dissection then proceeds in the subgaleal plane, between the galea and the pericranium, with the aid of a rhinoplasty lighted retractor and a 0° rigid

endoscope. The dissection is performed over the entire extent of the suture, from the anterior fontanelle to the nasofrontal suture. A ribbon retractor is often needed to obtain dissection in the most inferior portion where the nasofrontal suture is located.

A pediatric craniotome is then used to create a 7-mm burr hole at the incision site to access the dura. The burr hole is enlarged along the suture axis posteriorly using a 4- to 5-mm Kerrison rongeur. Once the suture is released from the burr hole to the anterior fontanel, a 30° rigid endoscope is advanced under the stenosed suture to develop the epidural space plane of dissection, which is then advanced to the nasofrontal suture. Careful attention is required approximately halfway down the forehead, where a prominent bridging vein often exists extending from the sagittal sinus. These veins can be a significant source of bleeding if not promptly cauterized, often performed using the endoscopic bipolar. The epidural plane must be dissected completely to the nasofrontal suture and anterior fontanelle. Once freed from the scalp and dura, a Mayo scissors, a pituitary rongeur, or a straight Leksell rongeur is used to cut a 4- to 5-mm strip of bone to the nasofrontal suture. Failure to do so will result in an unsuccessful correction.

Osseous hemostasis is performed throughout the case using a guarded Frasier tip suction, guarded ribbon retractors, and suction-cautery unit. Often, multiple passes are required for

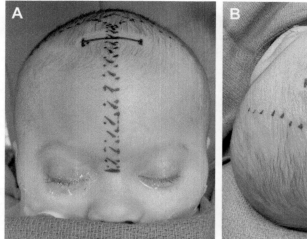
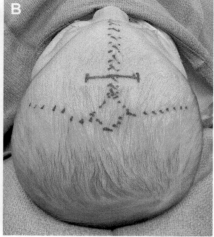

Fig. 11. Intraoperative markings for metopic synostosis. The 2.5-cm incision marking is made 1 to 2 cm behind the hairline; the dotted line represents the open bicoronal suture and anterior fontanel. The dashed line is the proposed craniectomy along the synostosed metopic suture, which is carried inferior to the nasofrontal suture. (*A*) Frontal view. (*B*) Bird's view.

complete hemostasis and can be performed until the bone is charred. Additional hemostasis is achieved using Surgiflo and liquid thrombin. The endoscope is reinserted, and the entire surgical field is closely inspected during a Valsalva maneuver for bleeding bridging veins, oozing diploe, or dural tears. The galea is closed with 4-0 Monocryl suture, and the skin is closed with Mastisol and Steri-Strips.

It should be noted that the dura overlying the metopic suture ossifies at a slower rate than over the vertex. Anterior growth of the brain also moves the frontal bone apart as much as 2 to 2.5 cm as can be seen on plain skull films postoperatively (**Fig. 12**). A large strip craniectomy can thus lead to large areas devoid of bone, and the osteotomy width should be limited to the width of the Kerrison rongeur. Following a successful surgery, compliance with helmet therapy and patience are the key to excellent results. Many times, complete resolution of the deformity is not appreciated until 2 to 4 years after the surgery; this is to be expected and is communicated to the parents preoperatively (**Fig. 13**).

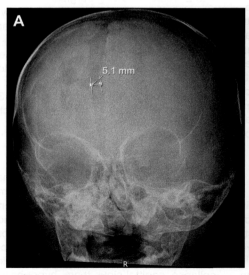
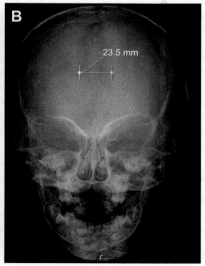

Fig. 12. Immediate postoperative and 12 months postoperative plain films demonstrating widening of metopic craniectomy. (*A*) Immediate postoperative image showing 4- to 5-mm craniectomy. (*B*) 12-months postoperative image demonstrating 18 to 19 mm of widening.

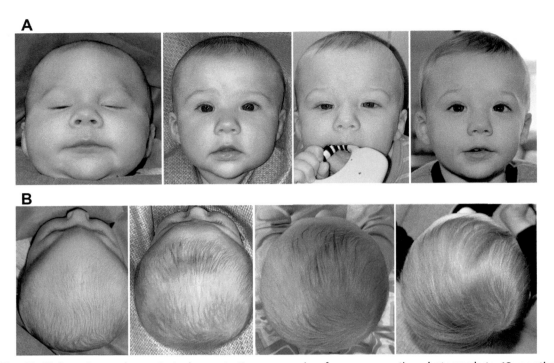

Fig. 13. Right unicoronal synostosis demonstrating progression from preoperative photograph to 12 months postoperatively. (*A*) Preoperative bird's view, 3 months, 6 months, 12 months, and 24 months postoperatively. (*B*) Preoperative bird's view, 3 months, 6 months, 12 months, and 24 months postoperatively.

POSTOPERATIVE CARE

Upon the conclusion of the procedure and removal of the endotracheal tube, patients stay overnight in the pediatric intensive care unit for observation. Pain is usually minimal and easily managed with oral acetaminophen and ibuprofen and with intravenous morphine for breakthrough pain. Patients generally begin oral intake shortly after the operation and are typically discharged the following morning. Nursing patients may breastfeed immediately upon the conclusion of surgery. Post-discharge pain control continues with scheduled, alternating doses of acetaminophen and ibuprofen every 3 hours for the next 3 days. Nearly all patients can be safely discharged on the first postoperative day.

HELMETS

Postoperative cranial orthotic helmet therapy is critical to the long-term success of endoscopic-assisted surgery. The helmet is fashioned on postoperative day 3 and delivered by postoperative day 5 following resolution of scalp swelling.[17] The helmet aids and guides in correcting the craniofacial deformity by applying pressure to areas of overgrowth and overcompensation (for example, the contralateral frontal bone in unicoronal synostosis), while providing extra space for areas of restricted growth secondary to craniosynostosis (such as the ipsilateral frontal bone). Changes to head shape may be seen as early as 1 to 2 weeks following surgical release.[43] Correction of the craniofacial deformity is a slow process, extending continuously for several years. Given cranial growth dynamics, the helmet must be worn at all times for 10 to 12 months after surgery or until approximately 1 year of age, following the end of the period of rapid brain growth[17] (**Fig. 14**).

Depending on the patient's age, 2 or 3 helmets may be necessary. Complete correction may take up to 4 years postoperatively.

DISCUSSION

Traditional open calvarial remodeling has meant delaying surgery until the infant is 9 months of age or older, followed by extensive bifrontal craniotomies and orbital bandeau remodeling.[20] Numerous complications have been documented, including coagulopathic states, hypotension, venous air embolism, dural tears, cardiovascular collapse, sagittal sinus tears, hypophosphatemia, hyponatremia, and residual calvarial defects.[17] Essentially 100% of patients require a blood

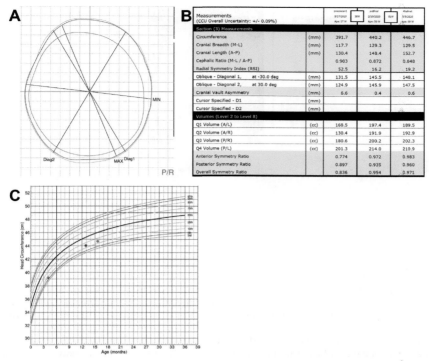

Fig. 14. Right unicoronal synostosis growth charts during postoperative helmet therapy. (*A*) Growth as directed by helmet therapy in the deficient area. (*B*) Significant improvement in all areas measured; it is especially important to note improvement in asymmetry indices. (*C*) Standard head growth chart; it is important to note that there is no cranial growth restriction secondary to helmet therapy. Head growth continues to follow curve as expected. CCU, ; Diag, diagnosis; MIN, minimum; MAX, maximum; P/R.

transfusion. Furthermore, careful analysis of the results has shown that the underlying deformational changes are often not adequately treated and become more and more apparent the further from surgery one is (**Fig. 15**).[9]

The endoscopic-assisted approach is a minimally invasive technique that uses the concept of open sutures and early propulsive growth of the brain, guided by active head molding using custom cranial orthotics.[1] The custom cranial orthotic helmets are critical to the success, as they counteract the tendency of the cranial vault to revert to the premorbid shape. The helmet is the difference from the failed simple suturectomy. This has resulted in excellent long-term results of the skull appearance and the facial skeleton in terms of correction of vertical dystopia, nasal deviation, craniofacial scoliosis, and maxillary and mandibular deformities in unicoronal cases, and hypotelorism in metopic cases. Time and patience are essential in these minimally invasive cases, as the full cosmetic result is often not fully appreciated until the child is more than 4 years after the surgery (**Fig. 16** and **17**).

Direct results comparisons are difficult, as there are no standard measurement systems. The most widely cited measurement strategies include anthropometry, CT, and 3-dimensional photogrammetry.[15,44,45] CT-based techniques are arguably the most precise, yet controversy exists given the need for radiation exposure and the lifetime oncologic risk.[46,47] Three-dimensional photogrammetry is reliable and interchangeable with CT.[48,49] There remains much controversy about the best points, angles, planes, indices, and proportions to use, resulting in minimal standardization.[15] There is undoubtedly a correlation between length of follow-up and worsening aesthetic results with open surgery.[38,50,51] Similarly, there is a correlation between length of follow-up and improving aesthetic results with early intervention using minimally invasive techniques. There has been a considerable time since the advent of endoscopic-assisted techniques, and no longer is long-term stability able to be legitimately questioned.[15,45]

Jimenez and Barone[20] used anthropometric measurements and photographic documentation to demonstrate the significant correction in most of their patients using endoscopic approaches. Among the 100 patients in their case series of unicoronal and metopic synostosis

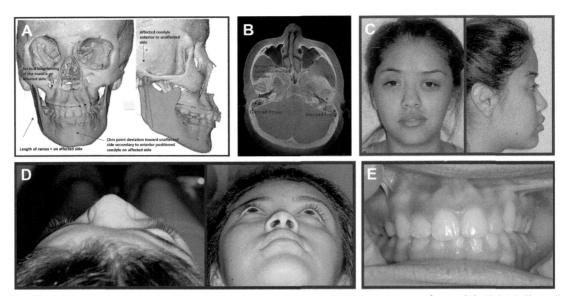

Fig. 15. A 20-year-old patient with right-sided coronal synostosis FOA at 1 year of age. (*A*) Right (affected) mandibular condyle anterior to left (unaffected). Chin point deviation to the unaffected side but clinical appearance toward unaffected side (refer to *C*). (*B*) Axial cut. Anterior displacement of the glenoid fossa, resulting in anterior displacement of the affected side condyle. Anterior projection of zygomaticomaxillary complex on the affected side. Although anteriorly projected hypoplastic when compared with the unaffected side. Gross overall appearance however is deficient on unaffected side. (*C*) Frontal and profile views. Significant relapse resulting in uncorrected appearance. Mandibular deviation, vertical dystopia, right supraorbital bar retraction, maxillary mandibular cant, nasal root, and tip deviation. (*D*) Bird's and worm's views. Supraorbital bar with significant retraction and temporal hollowing on affected side. Maxillary cant and yaw: despite hypoplastic maxilla on the right, left side appears more hypoplastic; this is secondary to yaw, but the appearance is deceiving. Mandible-chin point deviation toward unaffected side. (*E*) Occlusion. Maxillary cant down on the right 2 mm. Secondary to vertical elongation on ipsilateral side of mandibular ramus. Class I occlusion. Maxillomandibular complex contributing to overall facial asymmetry.

undergoing endoscopic-assisted repair, complications included 2 dural tears, 4 pseudomeningoceles, and 2 cases of incomplete reossification. The series showed that 84% of patients obtained excellent results, and 9% obtained good results. In the investigators' opinion, the cases of poor outcomes were secondary to noncompliance with cranial orthotics.

Although direct esthetic comparisons may be difficult, other surgical performance measures favor endoscopic-assisted craniosynostosis correction. A literature review comparing open and endoscopic techniques for metopic synostosis performed by Jimenez and colleagues14 found statistically significant results for age at the time of surgery (11.5 vs 3.8 months,

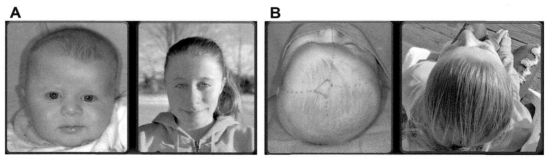

Fig. 16. Right unicoronal synostosis; long-term preoperative and postoperative photographs. (*A*) Right unicoronal synostosis preoperative frontal view and 12 years postoperative frontal view. (*B*) Bird's view preoperatively and 12 years postoperatively.

A

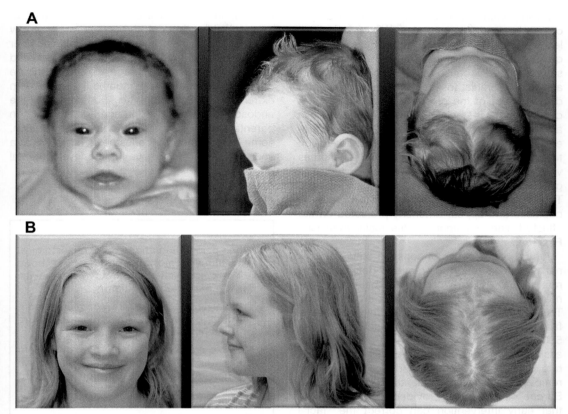

B

Fig. 17. Right unicoronal synostosis; long-term preoperative and postoperative photographs. (*A*) Metopic synostosis preoperative frontal, profile, and bird's view. (*B*) Metopic synostosis 9 years postoperatively frontal, profile, and bird's view.

P = .0089), mean EBL (224 vs 55.4 mL, P = .0003), mean operative time (223.7 vs 66.7 minutes, P = .0122), mean rate of transfusion (0.77 vs 0.22, P = .0028), and mean length of stay (3.7 vs 1.7 days, P = .0002).

Endoscopic-assisted coronal synostosis correction should ideally be performed on infants 3 months or younger and no older than 6 months,[20] although the upper limit is now being challenged. Correction of the associated deformity occurs faster when operated on at a younger age.[14] Nasal deviation correction begins to appear first and is usually fully corrected by 6 to 9 months postoperatively.[20] Next, the ipsilateral supraorbital rim moves forward with concurrent resolution of the associated proptosis. Over the next several years, as the brain continues to grow, the dystopic orbit descends. The last area to correct is the frontal plagiocephaly. The most beneficial result has been in resolving skull base changes, such as cranial scoliosis, thereby affecting maxillary and mandibular deformities, nasal deviation, and vertical dystopia. The procedure is associated with excellent results, no mortalities, and low morbidities. The instrumentation to perform the surgery is minimal and available in most hospitals.

Endoscopic-assisted metopic synostosis correction should be performed on patients under 12 weeks, although 8 weeks is ideal.[14] Good results are still seen between 3 and 6 months. Patients older than 6 months are not ideal candidates unless the presenting condition is very mild. In the case series of metopic synostosis correction, there were no cases of turricephaly. Turricephaly is common after open correction of metopic synostosis, in addition to various osseous defects along the edges of the osteotomies and where plates and screws once were.[14,38]

By waiting until 9 months or later to do an open repair, the correction targets only the anterior cranium and superior orbital rims. By doing so, open repairs neglect most of the orbital, nasal, maxillary, and mandibular deformities because the repair is performed after the cranial base is mostly determined. Early intervention before 8 months has been shown to decrease the progression and incidence of orbital and facial deformities secondary to the synostosis.[52–54]

It is important to understand that unicoronal synostosis begins in the central portion of the suture, leading to narrowing of the cranial base sphenosquamosal, sphenofrontal, and sphenoethmoidal sutures.[55–57] This causes shortening of the anterior and middle cranial fossae and results in anterior displacement of the glenoid fossa.[9] The consequence of this is "facial twisting," which results in a hypoplastic mandible with vertical ramus lengthening on the affected side and chin point deviation to the contralateral side. The maxilla becomes vertically hyperplastic on the affected side as it grows toward the mandible, resulting in a cant. The zygomaticomaxillary complex will also be hypoplastic and appear anteriorly projected on the affected side secondary to the facial twist (see **Fig. 15A**).

A study of 81 cases of nonsyndromic unicoronal synostosis reported an overall defect/relapse rate of 73% following frontal orbital advancement, with a total reoperation rate of 20%.[58] This study did not account for mid and lower face operations. Meanwhile, a recent study of 500 patients who underwent endoscopic-assisted surgeries found only a 2.8% reoperation rate, which further dropped to 1.2% when removing syndromic patients.[59] Jimenez and Barone[43] have also provided some evidence that early intervention can correct the "facial twist" with 88% of patients achieving at least a 70% correction and 77% of patients achieving a 100% correction. All patients who did not reach at least 70% correction were more than 8 months of age at the time of surgery.

Unlike traditional suturectomy, endoscopic-assisted repairs with postsurgical cranial orthotics have demonstrated at least equivalent results to open procedures in the correction of hypotelorism and other facial deformities.[60] Residual facial deformities from a metopic synostosis are generally minimal and usually related to the need for augmentation of the lateral orbital and bitemporal areas.[9] This is usually accomplished with cranial implants upon completion of cranial growth.

From a health care systems perspective, analysis and comparison of hospital charges for patients who underwent endoscopic-assisted approaches were approximately $14,000 versus roughly $39,000 in open calvarial vault remodeling.[14,17] The average helmet cost of $700 also far outweighed the cost of reoperation.

It should be noted that endoscopic techniques are not without their challenges. Metopic synostosis is often considered one of the more difficult synostosis patterns to treat endoscopically from a technical standpoint. These challenges include a small scalp incision, a relatively long distance from the incision to the endpoint of the suturectomy, working in and through a very narrow osteotomy, and the presence of a variable number of venous perforators.[14] The endoscopic-assisted technique is also limited by age and should only be offered to children over 9 months if they have an extremely mild deformity. Furthermore, the endoscopic-assisted approach does rely on parental compliance for the helmet. In addition, some have argued that anesthesia exposure at a younger age may have neurodevelopmental effects.[61]

CLINICS CARE POINTS

- When performing endoscopic craniectomies, meticulous hemostasis on bleeding bone edges is achieved throughout the case with the use of suction coagulators.
- Coronal craniectomies are completed from the anterior fontanel to the squamosal suture of the temporal bone.
- Metopic craniectomies are completed from the anterior fontanel to the nasofrontal junction but should be no more than 4 to 5 mm in width; otherwise, cranial defects may persist.
- The endoscopic bipolar is essential when performing metopic craniectomies, as it aids in coagulating emissary veins, which travel from the sagittal sinus to the skull and scalp.

REFERENCES

1. Jimenez DF, Barone CM. Endoscopic approach to coronal craniosynostosis. Clin Plast Surg 2004; 31(3):415–22.
2. Jimenez DF, Barone CM. Endoscopic technique for coronal synostosis. Child's Nervous Syst 2012;28: 1429–32.
3. van der Meulen J. Metopic synostosis. Childs Nerv Syst 2012;28:1359–67.
4. Lajeunie E, Le Merver M, Marchac D. Syndromal and nonsyndromal primary trigonocephaly: analysis of a series of 237 patients. Am J Med Genet 1998; 75:211.
5. Natghian H, Song M, Jayamohan J, et al. Long-term results in isolated metopic synostosis: the Oxford experience over 22 years. Plast Reconstr Surg 2018;142(4):509–15.
6. Keshavarzi S, Hayden MG, Ben-Haim S, et al. Variations of endoscopic and open repair of metopic craniosynostosis. J Craniofac Surg 2009;20(5): 1439–44.

7. Vu HL, Panchal J, Parker EE, et al. The timing of physiologic closure of the metopic suture: a review of 159 patients using reconstructed 3D CT scans of the craniofacial region. J Craniofac Surg 2001; 12(6):527–32.

8. Pindrik J, Molenda J, Uribe-Cardenas R, et al. Normative ranges of anthropometric cranial indices and metopic suture closure during infancy. J Neurosurg Pediatr 2016;25(6):667–73.

9. Yates, DM. The development, correction, and prevention of pathologic development secondary to craniosynostosis. In: Jimenez D, editor. Endoscopic craniosynostosis surgery. Elsevier; April 13, 2022:304.

10. Posnick JC, Lin KY, Chen P, et al. Metopic synostosis: quantitative assessment of presenting deformity and surgical results based on CT scans. Plast Reconstr Surg 1994;93(1):16–24.

11. Birgfeld CB, Saltzman BS, Hing AV, et al. Making the diagnosis: metopic ridge versus metopic craniosynostosis. J Craniofac Surg 2013;24(1):178–85.

12. McEwan TW, Martin AL, Tanaka T, et al. Evaluating children with metopic craniosynostosis: the cephalic width-intercoronal distance ratio. Cleft Palate Craniofac J 2016;53(4):95–100.

13. Anand A, Campion NJ, Cheshire J, et al. Analysis of cosmetic results of metopic synostosis: concordance and interobserver variability. J Craniofac Surg 2013;24(1):304–8.

14. Jimenez DF, McGinity MJ, Barone CM. Endoscopy-assisted early correction of single-suture metopic craniosynostosis: a 19-year experience. J Neurosurg Pediatr 2019;23:61–74.

15. Jaskolka M. Current controversies in metopic suture craniosynostosis. Oral Maxillofacial Surg Clin N Am 2017;29:447–63.

16. Cartwright CC, Jimenez DF, Barone CM, et al. Endoscopic strip craniectomy: a minimally invasive treatment for early correction of craniosynostosis. J Neurosci Nurs 2003;35:13–8.

17. Jimenez DF, Barone CM, Cartwright C, et al. Early management of craniosynostosis using endoscopic assisted strip craniectomies and cranial orthotic molding therapy. Pediatrics 2002;110:97–104.

18. Jimenez DF, Barone CM, McGee ME, et al. Endoscopy-assisted wide-vertex craniectomy, barrel stave osteotomies, and postoperative helmet molding therapy in the management of sagittal suture craniosynostosis. J Neurosurg Pediatr 2004;100:407–17.

19. Jimenez DF, Barone CM, McGee ME. Design and care of helmets in postoperative craniosynostosis patients: our personal approach. Clin Plast Surg 2004;31(3):481–7.

20. Jimenez DF, Barone CM. Early treatment of anterior calvarial craniosynostosis using endoscopic assisted minimally invasive techniques. Child's Nervous Syst 2007;23(12):1411–9.

21. Jimenez DF, Barone CM. Endoscopic assisted craniectomies for the management of craniosynostosis. In: Jimenez DF, editor. Neurosurgical topics: intracranial endoscopic neurosurgery. Park Ridge (IL): American Association of Neurological Surgeons; 1998. p. 209–20.

22. Jimenez DF, Barone CM. Endoscopic assisted wide vertex craniectomy, barrel stave osteotomies and postoperative helmet molding therapy in the early management of sagittal suture craniosynostosis. Neurosurg Focus 2000;9(3):E2.

23. Jimenez DF, Barone CM. Metopic synostosis. In: Benzel EC, Rengachary SS, editors. Calvarial and dural reconstruction. Park Ridge (IL): American Association of Neurological Surgeons; 1998. p. 135–40.

24. Jimenez DF, Barone CM. Endoscopic craniectomy for early surgical correction of sagittal craniosynostosis. J Neurosurg 1998;88:77–81.

25. Johnson JO, Jimenez DF, Barone CM. Blood loss after endoscopic strip craniectomy for craniosynostosis. J Neurosurg Anesthesiol 1999;12:60.

26. Johnson JO, Jimenez DF, Tobias JD. Anesthetic care during minimally invasive neurosurgical procedures in infants and children. Paediatr Anaesth 2002;12(6):478–88.

27. Knoll BI, Shin J, Persing JA. The bowstring canthal advancement: a new technique to correct the flattened supraorbital rim in unilateral coronal synostosis. J Craniofac Surg 2005;16:492–7.

28. Marchac D, Renier D, Broumand S. Timing of treatment for craniosynostosis and facio-craniosynostosis: a 20-year experience. Br J Plast Surg 1994;47:211–22.

29. Marsh JL, Schwartz HG. The surgical correction of coronal and metopic craniosynostoses. J Neurosurg 1983;59:245–51.

30. Ocal E, Sun PP, Persing JA. Craniosynostosis. In: Albright AL, editor. Principles and practice of pediatric neurosurgery. New York: Thieme; 2008. p. 265–88.

31. Persing J, Babler W, Winn HR, et al. Age as a critical factor in the success of surgical correction of craniosynostosis. J Neurosurg 1981;54:601–6.

32. Persing JA, Jane JA, Delashaw JB. Treatment of bilateral coronal synostosis in infancy: a holistic approach. J Neurosurg 1990;72:171–5.

33. Renier D, Brunet I, Marchac D. IQ and craniostenosis: evolution in treated and untreated cases. In: Marchac D, editor. Craniofacial surgery. Berlin (Germany): Springer-Verlag; 1987. p. 114–7.

34. Tobias JD, Johnson JO, Jimenez DF, et al. Venous air embolism during endoscopic strip craniectomy for repair of craniosynostosis in infants. Anesthesiology 2001;95:340–2.

35. Duke BJ, Mouchantat RA, Ketch LL, et al. Trans-cranial migration of microfixation plates and screws: case report. Pediatr Neurosurg 1996;25:31–4.

36. Joshi SM, Witherow H, Dunaway DJ, et al. The danger of using metallic plate and screw fixation in the young. Br J Neurosurg 2006;20:330.

37. Kosaka M, Myanohara T, Wada Y, et al. Intracranial migration of fixation wires following correction of craniosynostosis in an infant. J Craniomaxillofac Surg 2003;31(1):15–9.

38. Wes AM, Paliga JT, Goldstein JA, et al. An evaluation of complications, revisions, and long-term aesthetic outcomes in nonsyndromic metopic craniosynostosis. Plast Reconstr Surg 2014;133(6):1453–64.

39. Pelo S, Tamburrini G, Marianetti TM, et al. Correlations between the abnormal development of the skull base and facial skeleton growth in anterior synostotic plagiocephaly: the predictive value of a classification based on CT scan examination. Childs Nerv Syst 2011;27(9):1431–43.

40. Gasparini G, Saponaro G, Marianetti TM, et al. Mandibular alterations and facial lower third asymmetries in unicoronal synostosis. Childs Nerv Syst 2013;29(4):665–71.

41. Gociman B, Agko M, Blagg R, et al. Endoscopic-assisted correction of metopic synostosis. J Craniofac Surg 2013;24:763–8.

42. Jimenez DF, Barone CM. Endoscopic techniques in craniosynostosis. Atlas Oral Max Clin 2010;18(2):93–107.

43. Barone CM, Jimenez DF. Endoscopic craniectomy for synostosis. Plast Reconstr Surg 1999;104:1965–73.

44. Kolar JC, Salter EM. Preoperative anthropometric dysmorphology in metopic synostosis. Am J Phys Anthropol 1997;103(3):341–51.

45. Kung TA, Vercler CJ, Muraszko KM, et al. Endoscopic strip craniectomy for craniosynostosis: do we really underhand the indications, outcomes, and risks? J Craniofac Surg 2016;27(2):293–8.

46. Fearon JA, Singh DJ, Beals SP, et al. The diagnosis and treatment of single-sutural synostoses: are computed tomographic scans necessary? Plast Reconstr Surg 2007;120(5):1327–31.

47. Engel M, Castrillon-Oberndorfer G, Hoffmann J, et al. Value of preoperative imaging in the diagnostics of isolated metopic suture synostosis: a risk-benefit analysis. J Plast Reconstr Aesthet Surg 2012;65:1246–51.

48. McKay DR, Davidge KM, Williams SK, et al. Measuring cranial vault volume with three-dimensional photography: a method of measurement comparable to the gold standard. J Craniofac Surg 2010;21(5):1419–22.

49. Mendonca DA, Naidoo SD, Skolnick G, et al. Comparative study of cranial anthropometric measurement by traditional calipers to computed tomography and three-dimensional photogrammetry. J Craniofac Surg 2013;24(4):1106–10.

50. Sloan GM, Wells KC, Raffel C, et al. Surgical treatment of craniosynostosis: outcome analysis of 250 consecutive patients. Pediatrics 1997;100(1):E2.

51. Hansen M, Padwa BL, Scott RM, et al. Synostotic frontal plagiocephaly: anthropometric comparison of three techniques for surgical correction. Plast Reconstr Surg 1997;100(6):1387–95.

52. Jivraj BA, Schaeffer E, Bone JN, et al. A 24-month cost and outcome analysis comparing traditional fronto-orbital advancement and remodeling with endoscopic strip craniectomy and molding helmet in the management of unicoronal craniosynostosis: a retrospective bi-institutional review. JPRAS Open 2019;20:35–42.

53. MacKinnon S, Proctor MR, Rogers GF, et al. Improving ophthalmic outcomes in children with unilateral coronal synostosis by treatment with endoscopic strip craniectomy and helmet therapy rather than fronto-orbital advancement. J Aapos 2013;17(3):259–65.

54. Denis D, Genitori L, Bolufer A, et al. Refractive error and ocular motility in plagiocephaly. Childs Nerv Syst 1994;10(4):210–6.

55. Calandrelli R, D'Apolito G, Gaudino S, et al. Radiological assessment of skull base changes in children with syndromic craniosynostosis: role of "minor" sutures. Neuroradiology 2014;56(10):865–75.

56. Rogers GF. Discussion: cranioorbital morphology caused by coronal ring suture synostosis. Plast Reconstr Surg 2019;144(6):1414–5.

57. Rogers GF, Mulliken JB. Involvement of the basilar coronal ring in unilateral coronal synostosis. Plast Reconstr Surg 2005;115(7):1887–93.

58. Selber JC, Brooks C, Kurichi JE, et al. Long-term results following fronto-orbital reconstruction in nonsyndromic unicoronal synostosis. Plast Reconstr Surg 2008;121(5):251–60.

59. Riordan CP, Zurakowski D, Meier PM, et al. Minimally invasive endoscopic surgery for infantile craniosynostosis: a longitudinal cohort study. J Pediatr 2020;216:142–9.

60. Nguyen DC, Patel KB, Skolnick GB, et al. Are endoscopic and open treatments of metopic synostosis equivalent in treating trigonocephaly and hypotelorism? J Craniofac Surg 2015;26:129–34.

61. Backeljauw B, Holland SK, Altaye M, et al. Cognition and brain structure following early childhood surgery with anesthesia. Pediatrics 2015;136(1):1–12.

Management of Sagittal and Lambdoid Craniosynostosis
Open Cranial Vault Expansion and Remodeling

Michael R. Markiewicz, DDS, MPH, MD, FAAP, FRCD(c), FACS[a,b,c,d,]*,
Matthew J. Recker, MD[b], Renée M. Reynolds, MD[b]

KEYWORDS

- Craniosynostosis • Lambdoidal • Sagittal • Plagiocephaly • Craniofacial • Craniofacial dysostoses

KEY POINTS

- The treatment of single-suture craniosynostosis depends on patient-specific factors including suture involved, patient age, and parental preference.
- Patients older than 4 months are less likely to benefit from minimally invasive procedures such as endoscopic strip craniectomy and use of orthotics.
- Children between age 4 and 6 months with sagittal craniosynostosis are offered a modified pi-plasty.
- Children older than 6 months with sagittal craniosynostosis are offered cranial vault reconstruction focusing on posterior cranial vault expansion and remodeling.
- Patients with lambdoidal suture craniosynostosis older than 4 months are offered posterior cranial vault reconstruction.

INTRODUCTION: NATURE OF THE PROBLEM—SAGITTAL SYNOSTOSIS, OPEN EXPANSION, AND REMODELING

Craniosynostosis, which is in its simplest form is defined as a malformation in which one or more of the cranial sutures are prematurely fused, was first defined by Virchow in 1851.[1] In his report, Virchow described his observation of restricted growth perpendicular to the direction of the involved suture and compensatory overgrowth of the craniofacial vault parallel to it. More recent work has demonstrated that the phenotypical skull shapes of craniosynostosis result from of a complex pattern of compensatory growth of adjacent sutures.[2]

Sagittal synostosis, or the premature fusion of the sagittal suture, produces a scaphocephalic or dolichocephalic head shape (Fig. 1). Its prevalence is estimated at 1:2000 to 1:5000, with a 3:1 male-to-female predilection.[3] Following Virchow's law, growth ceases perpendicular to the fused suture causing bitemporal and biparietal narrowing. In addition, there is compensatory growth parallel to the involved suture, which leads to frontal and

a Department of Oral and Maxillofacial Surgery, School of Dental Medicine, University at Buffalo, Buffalo, New York, USA; b Department of Neurosurgery, Jacobs School of Medicine and Biomedical Sciences, Buffalo, New York, USA; c Divison of Pediatric Surgery, Department of Surgery, Jacobs School of Medicine and Biomedical Sciences, Buffalo, New York, USA; d Craniofacial Center of Western New York, John Oishei Children's Hospital, Buffalo, NY, USA
* Corresponding author. Department of Oral and Maxillofacial Surgery, School of Dental Medicine, University at Buffalo, Buffalo, New York, USA.
E-mail address: mrm25@buffalo.edu

Oral Maxillofacial Surg Clin N Am 34 (2022) 395–419
https://doi.org/10.1016/j.coms.2022.01.005
1042-3699/22/© 2022 Elsevier Inc. All rights reserved.

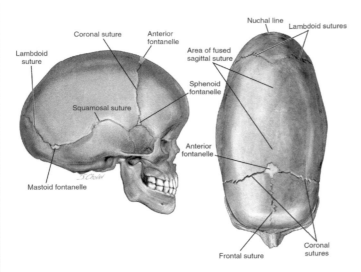

Coronal suture   Anterior fontanelle
Lambdoid suture
Area of fused sagittal suture
Sphenoid fontanelle
Squamosal suture
Anterior fontanelle
Mastoid fontanelle
Nuchal line   Lambdoid sutures
Frontal suture
Coronal sutures

Fig. 1. Lateral and bird's-eye views demonstrating scaphocephaly head shape with bitemporal and biparietal narrowing and anterior-posterior over-growth. *(From* Sinn DP, Dalton PS, and Tiwana PS. Chapter 44: Posterior Cranial Vault Remodeling. In: Kademani D, Tiwana PS,eds. Atlas of the Oral and Maxillofacial Surgery. 1st ed. Elsevier; 2016:453-461.)

occipital bossing. The result is the phenotypical long and thin skull shape.[1] There is variability in the degree of sutural involvement, with some patients only having a partial (anterior or posterior) fusion and some having complete fusion of the sagittal suture. Depending on the region of fusion along the suture, the anterior or posterior cranial vault can be predominantly affected.[3–7] If left untreated, potential consequences include continued cosmetic deformation, increased intracranial pressure and its associated sequelae, and neurodevelopmental delay. The incidence of neurodevelopmental delay in nonsyndromic single suture craniosynostosis ranges from 15%[8] to 37%[9] in some studies. The cause of neurodevelopmental delay remains poorly understood, but intrinsic central nervous system malformation and/or external compression of the brain by limited volume of the cranial vault are theorized to play a role.[10] Elevated intracranial pressure can occur due to the restriction in cranial volume expansion as the brain grows. Symptoms of raised intracranial pressure include headache, vomiting, and associated ophthalmologic findings including papilledema. Prolonged pressure on the optic nerves, when left untreated, can cause optic nerve neuropathy, atrophy, and blindness. Exotropia, strabismus, refractive errors, amblyopia, and exposure kerathopathy from exorbitism are also clinical findings.[11]

Lannelongue, in Paris, in 1890,[12] and then Lane, in San Francisco, in 1892,[13] were first credited with describing the management of sagittal suture craniosynostosis. In their initial reports, they both described only removal of the involved suture with no further management. Although these procedures did not directly correct the dysmorphology of the cranial vault, they remained a mainstay of care for nearly 7 decades. In

1967,[14,15] Tessier first described his innovative approach, which used a coronal incision to reconstruct the cranial vault and maxillofacial skeleton. Following Tessier's landmark reports, craniofacial surgery experienced a time of accelerated growth and innovation, with many advocating for early open reconstruction of the cranial vault for single-suture synostosis.[16,17]

The basic goals of contemporary surgical correction of craniosynostosis are to limit external brain compression from the cranial vault, improve head shape and aesthetics to ideal established norms, and to promote normal craniofacial growth and neurodevelopment.[18,19] The prevalence of lambdoid synostosis is far less than sagittal synostosis. Lambdoid synostosis will be addressed in the second half of this article.

INDICATIONS/CONTRAINDICATIONS FOR CORRECTION OF SAGITTAL SUTURE CRANIOSYNOSTOSIS

The authors' preferred timeline and hierarchy of procedures for correction of isolated sagittal suture craniosynostosis can be found in **Fig. 2.** The authors rarely perform anterior cranial vault expansion and remodeling (CVR)[20] or total CVR[21] for isolated sagittal suture craniosynostosis, as expansion of both the middle and posterior cranial vault in patients with all forms of sagittal synostosis has been shown to normalize forehead contour over time.[22] Additional treatment of the anterior cranial vault has been shown to be of minimal benefit.[20,23] An exception to this would be in an older child with significant frontal bossing where the calvarium is not as malleable and brain growth has decelerated or in the syndromic patient. The

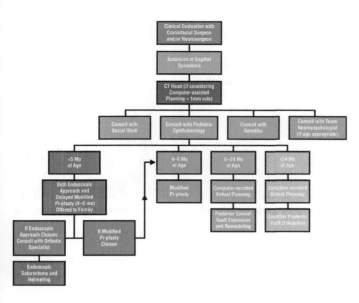

Fig. 2. Flow diagram for the authors' preferred management of isolated sagittal craniosynostosis.

authors follow a different paradigm for syndromic or multisuture craniosynostosis involving the sagittal suture, which is discussed elsewhere in this text. Indications and contraindications for repair of isolated sagittal suture craniosynostosis are presented in **Table 1**.

For patients presenting with isolated sagittal synostosis, treatment options include endoscopic and open techniques. Selection of surgical approach depends on multiple factors including patient age, medical comorbidities, and parental preference.

For patients presenting at an early age, endoscopic strip craniectomy and helmeting can be offered (see **Fig. 2**). Evidence suggests that patients may be effectively treated with endoscopic strip craniectomy up to 6 months of age.[24] The benefits of an endoscopic approach include less operative time, reduced blood loss, and decreased hospital length of stay. Endoscopic assisted correction of sagittal suture craniosynostosis is discussed in Shakir and colleagues' article, "Management of Sagittal and Lambdoid Craniosynostosis: Minimally Invasive Approaches," of this text. Patients who undergo intervention at a later age are less likely to have a successful outcome from an endoscopic strip craniectomy, and thus an "open" approach is favored. In our practice, an endoscopic approach is offered only to patients younger than 5 months. In these patients, the risks and benefits of both an endoscopic and "open" approach are discussed with the family. If the parents prefer an "open" approach but the child is too young, they may elect to wait until the child is old enough for an "open" procedure. The authors' preference is to wait until 4 months of age to perform an "open" reconstruction. For patients 4 to 6 months of age, a modified pi-plasty is offered, and therefore this procedure will be highlighted in this text.[25] The use of sagittal springs for spring-assisted expansion will not be discussed;

Table 1		
Indications and contraindications for repair of isolated sagittal suture craniosynostosis		
Indications	**Contraindications**	
Neurodevelopmental delay	Other causes for developmental delay	
Concern for increased intracranial pressure	Medically unstable or unable to undergo general anesthesia	
Abnormal head shape	—	
Exophthalmos or exorbitism	—	
Evidence of papilledema, optic nerve atrophy, or loss of vision	—	

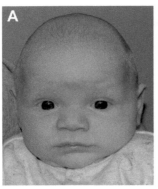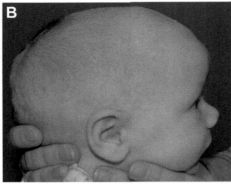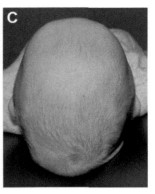

Fig. 3. Frontal (*A*), side (*B*), and bird's-eye (*C*) views of a 2-month-old demonstrating the characteristic findings of isolated sagittal synostosis.

however, this approach has been found to be successful in patients 3 to 6 months of age.[26,27]

TECHNIQUE/PROCEDURE FOR SAGITTAL SUTURE CRANIOSYNOSTOSIS
Modified Pi-plasty

Preoperative planning
The patient initially meets with the Pediatric Craniofacial, Neurosurgery, Ophthalmology, and Genetics teams. If warranted and age appropriate, the patient will meet with the team's neuropsychologist. At this time the cranial vault is examined, and a preliminary diagnosis is made (**Fig. 3**). Cranial imaging is obtained to confirm the diagnosis. A computed tomography (CT) scan is preferred over radiography, and it will be used for preoperative planning and postoperative comparisons (**Fig. 4**).

Preparation and patient positioning
1. The patient is placed supine onto the operating room table. Following the induction of general anesthesia, an oral endotracheal tube is placed and secured to the patient's midline. Two large bore peripheral venous access lines and an arterial line for intraoperative blood pressure monitoring are placed by the anesthesia team. A foley catheter is placed. Blood products are confirmed to be available, and tranexamic acid is frequently given perioperatively to reduce blood loss. Although it is not routine at our institution, some centers use a central venous catheter and precordial Doppler.

2. Often the authors will mark the incision before positioning the patient prone such that facial features can be visualized and placement can be optimized (**Fig. 5**). A curvilinear wavy incision is preferred and for men, this is marked so that the peaks of the waves coincide with the shape of hair recession seen with male pattern baldness:
   • Anterior peak at midline
   • Posterior peaks at temporal lines
   • Once the marking is satisfactory, a small 2 cm width of hair is clipped along the proposed coronal incision.

3. A preauricular or postauricular extension is seldomly used, as this is not found to be needed in the setting of a modified pi-plasty, and

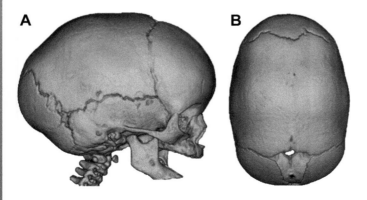

Fig. 4. Lateral (*A*) and bird's-eye (*B*) views of preoperative CT of the patient with isolated sagittal synostosis.

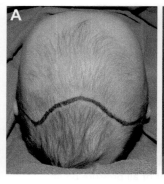
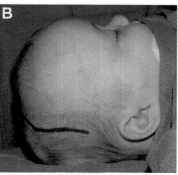

Fig. 5. Bird's-eye (*A*) and lateral (*B*) views demonstrating incision placement. Incision follows pattern of potential male pattern baldness, is posterior to the superficial temporal vessels, and has postauricular vector.

avoidance of this extension helps to optimize the chances of an inconspicuous and esthetic scar. If caudal extension of the incision is needed, it is done in the postauricular, rather than preauricular direction.

- Attention is taken to mark the incision posterior to the superficial temporal vessels, which are usually visualized through the skin in this age group. This technique will spare them during incision and dissection.

4. The incision and surrounding area are infiltrated with 0.5% Lidocaine with 1:200,000 epinephrine.

5. Meticulous care is taken to avoid any direct pressure on the patient's eyes. Foam padding with cut-outs for the eyes is applied before the patient being positioned prone (**Fig. 6**).

6. Before flipping the patient to a prone position, the direction of rotation and security of the patient must be discussed and coordinated between the anesthesia, surgery, and nursing teams. The patient's head and body need to be supported so that they are aligned in a neutral position during flipping and once prone. After lifting the patient, and before positioning prone, gel rolls and padding are placed at all pressure points including the chest, abdomen, and thighs bilaterally. The patient is then positioned prone in a Mayfield horseshoe headrest.

The cervical spine should be in a neutral position (**Fig. 7**).

7. The patient's eyes are inspected by looking through the Mayfield horseshoe headrest to visually confirm that no pressure is on the globe. In addition, the lateral orbital rims should be palpated to confirm that the orbits are not in contact with the head rest. The anesthesia, neurosurgery, and craniofacial teams should each examine the eyes for any pressure after positioning.[28]

8. Before the formal prep, the head, including the ears and exposed face, are thoroughly cleaned with 10 chlorhexidine-soaked sponges, followed by 10 alcohol-soaked sponges, and then thoroughly dried. The patient is then formally prepped with betadine paint solution. The surgical site is draped with towels followed by a craniotomy drape.

SURGICAL APPROACH

1. A skin incision is made along the marking described earlier with a 15 blade scalpel down to the deep dermis (**Fig. 8**). Two double-prong Guthrie skin hooks are used to apply gentle tension away from the incision while elevating the tissues. Sharp dissection through dermis, subcutaneous tissue, and

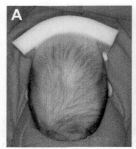
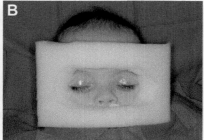
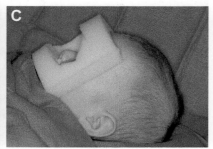

Fig. 6. Bird's-eye (*A*), frontal (*B*), and side (*C*) views demonstrating padding to protect eyes.

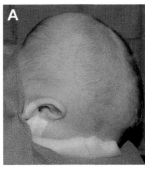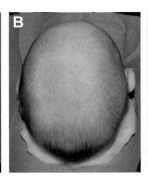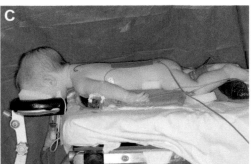

Fig. 7. (*A, B*) Padding once patient is flipped. (*C*) Padding of the body with relief of all pressure points.

galea aponeurotica is performed using a monopolar Bovie electrocautery with a Colorado needle tip (**Fig. 9**).

2. Dissection is taken down to the suprapericranial/subgaleal plane.
3. This is repeated along the length of the marked incision in 5 to 7 cm increments with meticulous hemostasis to minimize blood loss (**Fig. 10**). The authors do not use Raney clips, as they find they are unnecessary and create tissue trauma.
4. Once the subgaleal plane is dissected along the entirety of the incision, a rapid and relatively bloodless dissection is taken anterior and posterior exposing all areas of the proposed craniotomy including rostral to the coronal sutures, caudal to the external occipital protuberance, and inferior to the squamosal suture. The pericranium is left attached to the calvarium without dissection of the subpericranial plane (**Fig. 11**).

SURGICAL PROCEDURE

Step 1: the sites of the craniotomy and barrel staves for the modified pi-plasty are scored and marked with monopolar electrocautery and are illustrated in **Fig. 12**.

Step 2: the anterior fontanelle is usually patent and if feasible can be used to access the subdural space anteriorly for the craniotomy. If not feasible due to its size, an anterior burr hole is created just posterior to the fontanelle bilaterally approximately 1 cm lateral to the fused sagittal suture. Two to three additional pairs of parasagittal burr holes are then made posteriorly along the sagittal suture. This plane corresponds to the planned superior aspect of the lateral barrel staves (**Fig. 13**). All burr holes are created using an Acorn drill bit to create a small central opening at the burr hole site. The burr holes are expanded using a small curette and 2 mm Kerrison until a Penfield #3 elevator can be placed within each burr hole. The Penfield #3 is then used to strip the dura from the overlying cranium between each burr hole site on either side of the sagittal suture (**Fig. 14**). This release helps to prevent the creation of a dural tear during the craniotomy.

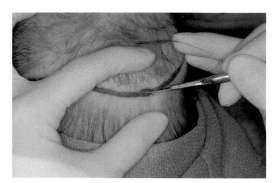

Fig. 8. Skin incision through epidermis with 15 blade.

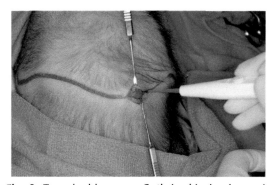

Fig. 9. Two double-prong Guthrie skin hooks apply gentle tension away from the incision while elevating the tissues, whereas dermis, subcutaneous, and galea aponeurotica layers are sharply dissected.

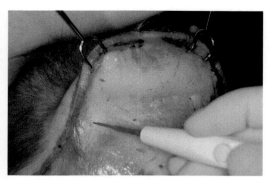

Fig. 10. A bloodless subgaleal plane is sharply dissected.

- Once the dura has been freed, a pediatric footplate is used to make 2 parasagittal cuts connecting the burr holes on either side of the sagittal suture from anterior to posterior. Care is taken to respect the 1 cm distance from midline to avoid risk to the superior sagittal sinus.
- Once complete, the Penfield #3 is used to release the dura across the midline at the anterior burr hole sites. Care must be taken to avoid injury to the superior sagittal sinus; although in the setting of a prematurely fused suture, the dura overlying the sinus is typically not found to be adherent. The Penfield #3 is kept in position across midline, whereas the pediatric footplate is again used to release the sagittal suture anteriorly.
- The sagittal suture is then slowly elevated away from the underlying dura under direct visualization until the posterior most set of burr holes are reached. Any dural bleeding is immediately addressed with Bipolar cautery. In addition, a large rectangular piece of gelfoam soaked in thrombin and a one-half by

3 cm patty is placed along the superior sagittal sinus to protect it from injury during the remaining aspects of the case.
- Approximately 5 to 6 barrel stave osteotomies are then planned from just anterior to the coronal sutures to just anterior to the lambdoid sutures bilaterally. The staves start from the previously elevated sagittal suture segment and extend laterally to just below the level of the squamosal suture (**Fig. 15**). During the barrel stave creation the assistant uses a suction and Penfield #1 to dissect and retract the dura under direct visualization, whereas the primary surgeon uses the pediatric footplate to fashion the cuts. Care must be taken to fully release the coronal sutures, which are generally adherent to the underlying dura given their patency.
- Following the barrel stave creation, the dura is freed in similar fashion along the bilateral lambdoid sutures and the occipital regions. Osteotomies are then carried from the midline sagittal segment across the lambdoid suture and laterally in parallel with the posterior most barrel stave. This cut is then turned posteriorly and medially along the inferior occipital region stopping approximately 1 cm from the external occipital protuberance.
- Once complete, the midline and occipital regions are secured only through the small residual midline bone segment at the external occipital protuberance. The frontal and parietal barrel staves remain secured to the temporal bone.

Step 3: following completion of all osteotomies, a broad-tipped tonsil forceps is used to bend the frontal and parietal barrel staves (**Fig. 16**A–C) to create a greenstick fracture at their base. The surgeon should hear or

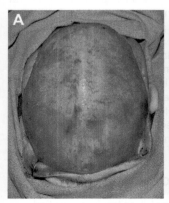 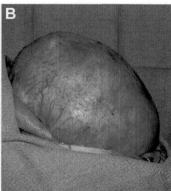

Fig. 11. Bird's-eye (A) and lateral (B) views of cranial vault exposed in subgaleal plane demonstrating vascularized pericranium.

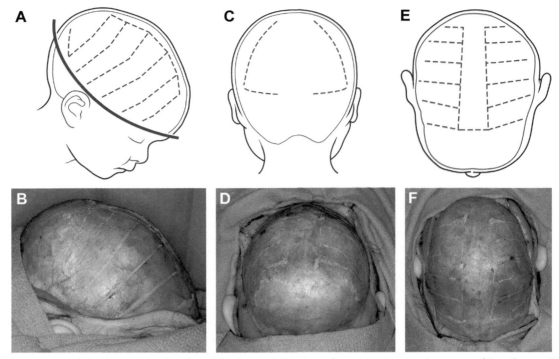

Fig. 12. Lateral (*A, B*), posterior (*C, D*), and bird's-eye (*E, F*) views demonstrating craniotomy markings for modified pi-plasty.

feel when the fracture is created, taking care to not complete the fracture leaving only the overlying periosteum as an attachment. This is then repeated along all the barrel staves.

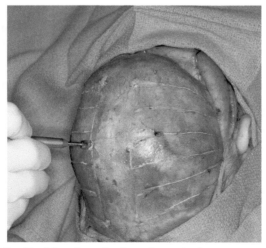

Fig. 13. A burr is made along the sagittal suture corresponding to the superior aspect of the planned lateral barrel staves.

Step 4: the occipital segments are subsequently fractured with the same technique (**Fig. 16**D)

Step 5: Tessier bone bending forceps are then used to microfracture, shape, and contour the barrel staves until they are malleable (**Fig. 17**A).

Step 6: a Leksell rongeur is used to trim sharp edges along the medial barrel staves and any additional areas that may overlap (**Fig. 17**B).

Step 7: to accommodate the anterior-posterior shortening created when the sagittal suture is released, the anterior aspect of the central sagittal segment is trimmed 1 to 2 cm. The barrel staves should not be overlapping (**Fig. 18**)

Step 8: the wound is irrigated with copious amounts of normal saline.

Step 9: closure is initiated with multiple deep inverted interrupted 3-0 Vicryl sutures. Attention is made to include galea aponeurotica and dermis in the deep closure. Skin closure takes place with a running 4-0 Vicryl Rapide suture (**Fig. 19**).

IMMEDIATE POSTOPERATIVE CARE

- Antibiotic ointment (bacitracin) is applied.

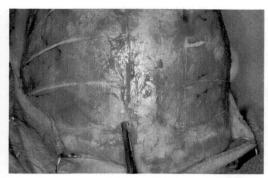

Fig. 14. Penfield #3 is then used to strip the dura from the overlying cranium between each burr hole site on either side of the sagittal suture.

- The authors do not routinely place drains for cranial vault remodeling procedures. The hair is washed with warm saline.
- The patient is carefully flipped over back to the supine position. Careful attention is made not to dislodge the endotracheal tube.
- The authors do not routinely place a headwrap.
- The patient is extubated and admitted to the intensive care unit.

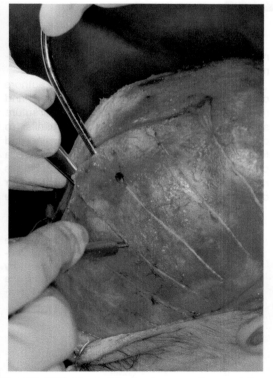

Fig. 15. With the assistant using a suction and Penfield #1 to dissect and retract the dura under direct visualization, the primary surgeon uses the pediatric footplate to fashion the cuts.

- Because there is little to no periorbital dissection, periorbital edema is generally not significant enough to cause eye closure, although this is occasionally encountered.
- Feeding and normal care resumes that night.
- Antibiotic ointment is applied for a minimum of 3 days.
- The wound is cleaned of scabs and debris once daily using a mix of half peroxide and half normal saline.
- Mild baby shampoo is used once a day, starting on postoperative day 3 to clean the head and wound. The wound may not be submerged for 2 weeks postoperatively.

INTERMEDIATE AND LONG-TERM POSTOPERATIVE CARE

- The patient is usually transferred to surgical floor status on postoperative day 1 to 2.
- Most patients are discharged on postoperative day 3 to 4. The patient is deemed ready for discharge when they are tolerating adequate oral intake, pain is controlled with oral medications, and spontaneous eye opening has returned if there was significant periorbital edema.
- Incision care is as described previously.
- The patient is seen at 2 weeks and 6 weeks postoperatively (**Fig. 20**A–C), then at 3 months (**Fig. 20**D–F), then at 1 year, and yearly thereafter.
- A CT will be taken in the immediate postoperative period to serve as a baseline for craniofacial appearance and dimensions (**Fig. 20**G–I); this is also to confirm adequate spacing with no overlap of the bony segments.
- The patient sees pediatric ophthalmology every year for a fundoscopic examination to assess for papilledema and any signs of increased intracranial pressure. When indicated, the patient is referred and managed by the team neuropsychologist who will assess for any signs of neurodevelopmental delay.

POTENTIAL COMPLICATIONS AND MANAGEMENT

Table 2 lists potential compilations and their management.

Technique/Procedure for Sagittal Suture Craniosynostosis

Cranial vault remodeling
After 6 months of age, the authors prefer open CVR. The authors do not prefer one particular

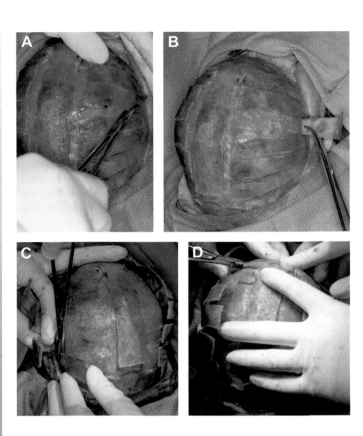

Fig. 16. A tonsil forceps is used to green-stick fracture and bend the barrel staves (A–C); this is then performed on the occipital segment (D).

approach to open CVR, rather a customized approach matching the procedure to the deformity, which may include a variety of procedures such as switch cranioplasty,[29] Hung span,[30] or even distraction osteogenesis for those at advanced age. Fig. 21 illustrates multiple potential reconstructions for a 2-year-old patient with sagittal synostosis. The authors' approach is to assess potential virtual operative plans and choose the operation that will achieve normal anthropometric measurements and normal morphologic appearance for the child, while promoting normal future craniofacial growth.

Other than in unique circumstances, the authors opt for posterior cranial vault expansion and remodeling. In the case of complete sagittal suture synostosis, our experience has been similar to others in that we have found frontal bossing and forehead deformities to resolve over time after a posterior CVR.[22] Total cranial vault remodeling is rarely necessary in this age group.[22] As with other operations for sagittal suture craniosynostosis, the

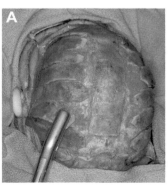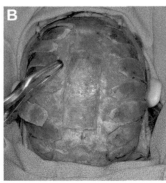

Fig. 17. Tessier bone bending forceps are used to microfracture, shape, and contour the barrel staves (A), followed by trimming of any sharp edges along the medial barrel staves with a Leksell rongeur (B).

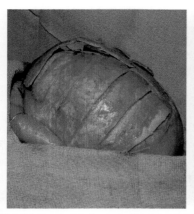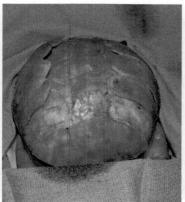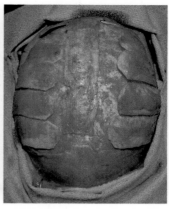

Fig. 18. Lateral (*A*), posterior (*B*), and bird's-eye (*C*) view of cranial vault before closure.

ultimate goal of this procedure is to increase the bitemporal and biparietal width and decrease the anterior-posterior length of the cranial vault.

PREOPERATIVE PLANNING

Preoperative planning for open CVR is similar to that described for a modified pi-plasty.
- Initial consultation and discussion with both Craniofacial and Neurosurgery teams (**Fig. 22**A, B).
- A CT of the head is obtained (**Fig. 22**C, D). The CT serves as an aid in diagnosis and is necessary for computer-assisted virtual planning. The authors do no routinely use virtual planning for endoscopic or modified pi-plasty procedures.
- When using virtual computer planning, the CT scan is completed using specific specifications (matrix of 512 × 512 at 0.625 mm slice thickness, 25 cm or lesser field-of-view, 0° gantry tilt, and 1:1 pitch). It is important to note that a slice thickness of 0.625 mm is advised; however, larger slice spacing may be adequate depending on the application.
- The DICOM-formatted CT images are then transferred to the appropriate surgical planning software or third-party engineer and planner.
- Virtual computer planning session is performed with a goal of establishing normal cranial dimensions. Surgical craniotomies are marked and segmented and manipulated to an ideal position (**Fig. 23**).

Preparation and Patient Positioning

1. Patient preparation and positioning is similar to that described previously. For CVR, the post-auricular aspect of the incision is marked more inferior than for more minimal approaches, but this inferior extent is seldom needed during surgery, as subgaleal undermining and retraction allow for a smaller incision and approach (**Fig. 24**A, B).

Surgical Approach

The incision is marked as previously described (see **Fig. 24**A, B). A subgaleal dissection is performed (**Fig. 24**C, D).

Step 1: in contrast to the modified pi-plasty previously described, this procedure is carried

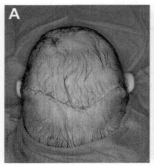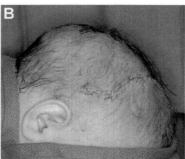

Fig. 19. Bird's-eye (*A*) and lateral (*B*) views just after skin closure.

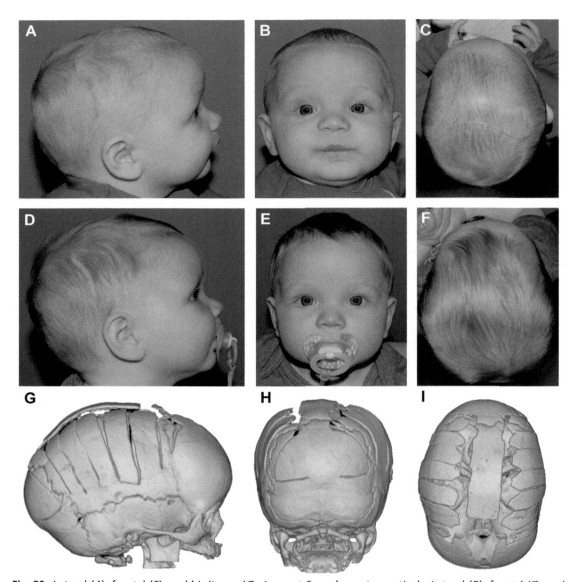

Fig. 20. Lateral (*A*), frontal (*B*), and bird's-eye (*C*) views, at 6 weeks postoperatively. Lateral (*D*), frontal (*E*), and bird's-eye (*F*) views, at 3 months postoperatively, demonstrating decreased anterior-posterior length and appropriate bitemporal and biparietal widening. Lateral (*G*), posterior (*H*), and bird's-eye (*I*) views of a 3-dimensional (3D) reconstructed CT taken in the immediate postoperative period.

out in the subpericranial plane. Accordingly, the pericranium and temporalis muscles are marked for incision and reflection, which includes incisions at the superior temporal lines bilaterally (blue) and at the approximate area of the posterior fontanelle, which is taken inferiorly to below the level of the squamosal suture (green) (**Fig. 24**E). Anteriorly and posteriorly based pericranial flaps are reflected. Bilateral inferiorly based temporalis flaps are reflected.

Step 2: judicious use of bone wax is used to address any bony oozing.

Surgical Procedure

Step 1: the cutting guide is applied to the cranial vault, and the craniotomy lines are marked with a sterile pencil (**Fig. 25**A, B).

Step 2: the neurosurgery team then completes the craniotomies, and the cranial vault is removed (**Fig. 25**C, D). The lateral parietal segments and middle sagittal suture segment

Table 2
Potential compilations and their management

Complication	Management
Poor wound healing	With proper incision care (see earlier discussion), wound complications are rare. However, the increased cranial volume places significant stress on the incision line, which can lead to dehiscence. Local wound care is typically the first step if dehiscence is focal and without signs of infection, although occasionally a return to the operating room for wound revision is necessary.
Surgical site infection	This is rare in this population and may be managed with local wound care, antibiotics, and sometimes surgical washout.
Corneal abrasion	The best management is prevention by properly dressing the eyes with semiocclusive dressings and thorough washing of the globes with a balance salt solution at the conclusion of the case. Management of a corneal abrasion includes ophthalmology consultation and antibiotic ointment to prevent scarring.
Dural tear and associated cerebrospinal fluid (CSF) leak	The best management is prevention with thorough dural release and protection before making the surgical cuts. Even in the setting of a dural tear intraoperatively a postoperative CSF leak is very rare with meticulous closure of any dural lacerations/tears. In the case of a postoperative CSF leak, otorrhea and/or rhinorrhea would not be expected, as no orbital or mastoid osteotomies are created. A CSF leak would typically present as a subgaleal pseudomeningocele or frank CSF leakage from the incision. Management can include oversewing of the wound, maintaining upright positioning, pseudomeningocele tap for drainage, CSF diversion by placement of a temporary lumbar drain, open surgical repair, or in rare cases placement of a ventriculoperitoneal shunt.
Venous air embolism (VAE)	The is a rare but potentially fatal complication. It can potentially be detected by use of a precordial Doppler ultrasonic probe or transesophageal echocardiography. When it occurs findings include sudden and profound hypotension. The most fatal complication is cardiovascular collapse. Signs include sudden drop in the end tidal CO_2 followed quickly by hypotension and bradycardia. Treatment of VAE is aimed at stopping the inflow of air into the venous circulation and managing any complications that may arise. • Immediately irrigate the field copiously to prevent further air entry • If able, wax any exposed bone and repair any vascular defect • Use 100% oxygen, avoid nitrous oxide Initiate high-rate IV fluids • The head of the patient should be lowered to the level of the right atrium • If possible, place patient in left lateral decubitus position (Durant maneuver) • If central venous catheter is in place, attempt to aspirate air • If cardiovascular collapse is present ACLS/PALS should be followed • Use hyperbaric oxygen therapy, if available

(continued on next page)

Table 2
(continued)

Complication	Management
Need for postoperative blood transfusion	This is not a complication, as transfusion is expected in most open cranial vault remodeling procedures. However, the need for additional postoperative blood transfusion can potentially be avoided by appropriately typing and cross-matching patients, and transfusing during surgery, as well as judicious use of bone wax for bony bleeding, and use of monopolar and bipolar electrocautery to obtain soft tissue hemostasis.
Sagittal sinus tear	This is a rare but potentially life-threatening complication. Prevention is key with gentle release of the overlying dura before using the drill and protection of the sinus throughout the case. If a tear occurs, anesthesia should be immediately notified as the patient can lose significant amounts of blood quickly. Immediate attempts at repair should be made by suturing and coagulating gelfoam over the torn segment. If this is unable to stop the hemorrhage and the patient is in critical condition the sinus may be closed off using nurolon sutures, although this should be a last resort, as severe venous infarctions can result.

are taken to the back table (**Fig. 25**E). Evidence of increased intracranial pressure can be seen on the inner table of the calvarium (**Fig. 25**F).

Step 3: the bony segments are then switched to the contralateral side and applied along with the sagittal suture segment to the bony repositioning guide (**Fig. 25**G). Bone wax can be used to stabilize the segments on the guide.

Step 4: barrel staves are applied to the occipital segment, and it is flattened with the Tessier bone benders to reduce occipital bossing and anterior-posterior length.

Step 5: the occipital segment is applied to the guide, and it is secured along with the other segments using resorbable poly-D,L-lactic acid (PDLLA)/poly-L-lactic acid (PLLA) fixation (**Fig. 25**H, I).

Step 6: the reconstructed complex is then transferred over to the patient and fixed with PDLLA/PLLA resorbable fixation (**Fig. 25**J–L).

Step 7: split calvarial bone grafts are applied to all critically sized calvarial defects.

Step 8: careful attention and time is spent reapproximating the pericranial flaps and temporalis muscles. This is done using simple interrupted 3-0 Vicryl sutures (**Fig. 26**A–C). This is critical to prevent temporal hollowing.

Step 9: closure of the galea aponeurotica and skin is performed in the same manner as described previously (**Fig. 26**D).

Immediate Postoperative Care

- This is similar to that previously described for modified pi-plasty.

Intermediate and Long-Term Postoperative Care

- Intermediate and postoperative care is similar to that described previously. The patient is again seen 2 (**Fig. 27**A–C) and 6 weeks postoperatively, followed by 3 months, then 1 year (**Fig. 27**D, E), and yearly there after (**Fig. 27**F–H). A CT is obtained in the first 48 hours and then 1 year after surgery (**Fig. 27**I).

Possible Complications and Management

- Similar to that described previously for the modified pi-plasty procedure
- With CVR, given the patient's age, there is a higher chance of contour deformities, residual cranial vault defects, and the potential need for additional procedures. This is rare and can be addressed with cranioplasty.
- Fixation can fail, although this is rare. The management would be to return to the operating room and to refixate unstable bone segments.
- Closure can be difficult in large cranial expansions; this can be remedied by subgaleal dissection on approach. If a subperiosteal approach is used, the pericranium can be scored for released.
- If possible, fixation hardware should not be positioned underneath the incision, as this can cause increased stress on the incision and possibly erosion of hardware through the wound.

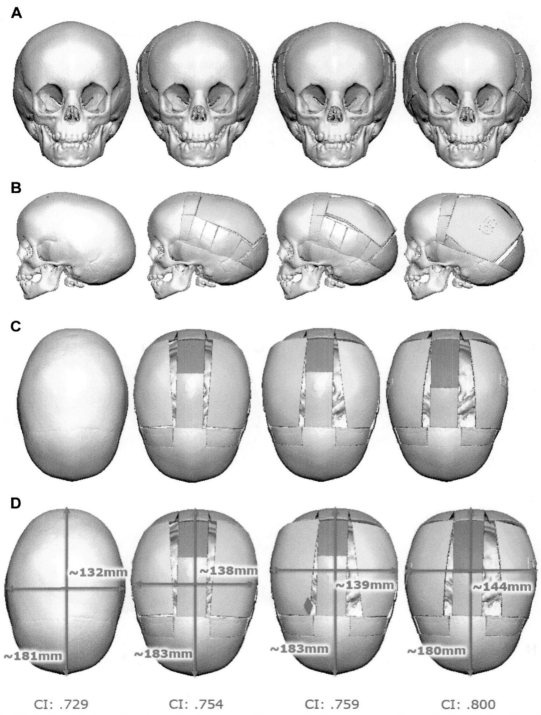

CI: .729   CI: .754   CI: .759   CI: .800

Fig. 21. (*A*)Frontal views of various virtual reconstructions. Left to right are the native patient cranial vault, a virtual Hung span cranioplasty, a virtual Hung span cranioplasty with switching of the parietal segments, and a switch cranioplasty. Fig. 21B illustrates lateral views, and Fig. 21C demonstrates bird's-eye views along with cranial measurements of proposed plans (*D*).

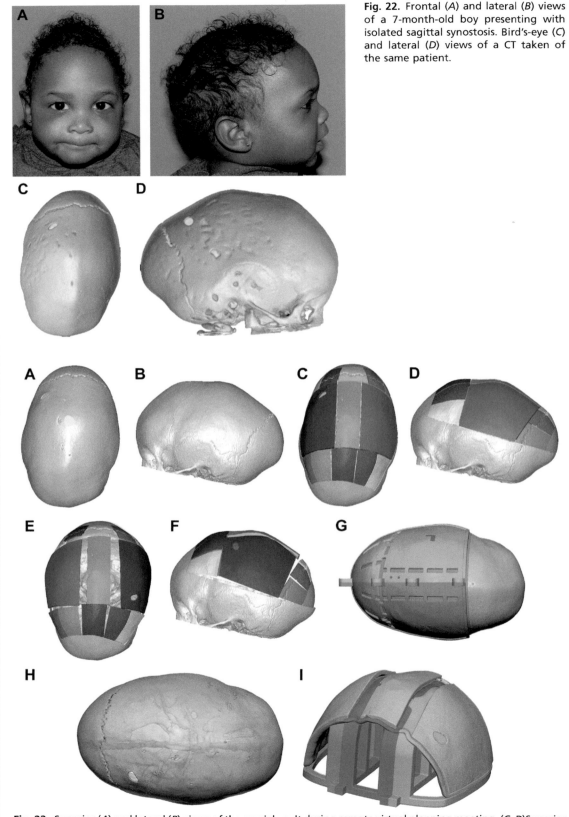

Fig. 22. Frontal (*A*) and lateral (*B*) views of a 7-month-old boy presenting with isolated sagittal synostosis. Bird's-eye (*C*) and lateral (*D*) views of a CT taken of the same patient.

Fig. 23. Superior (*A*) and lateral (*B*) views of the cranial vault during remote virtual planning meeting. (*C, D*)Superior and lateral views of the segmented cranial vault. The same views demonstrate proposed switch cranioplasty for cranial vault remodeling and expansion (*E, F*). (*G*)The proposed virtual cutting guide. (*H*) A virtual representation of the sagittal sinus. (*I*) A virtual representation of the positioning guide for the cranial segments (for use of external plating).

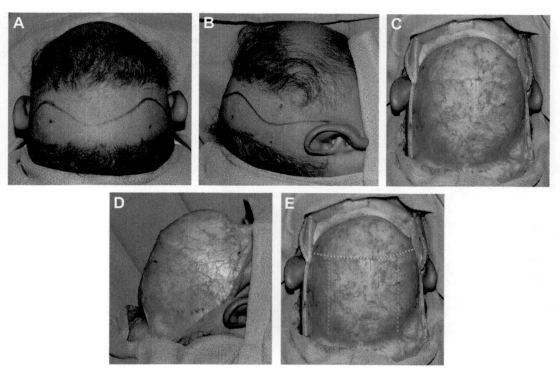

Fig. 24. (*A, B*) Bird's-eye and lateral views of the incision marking with patient positioned prone. (*C, D*) Bird's-eye and lateral views after subgaleal exposure. (*E*) Markings for anteriorly and posteriorly based pericranial flaps and bilateral inferiorly based temporalis flaps.

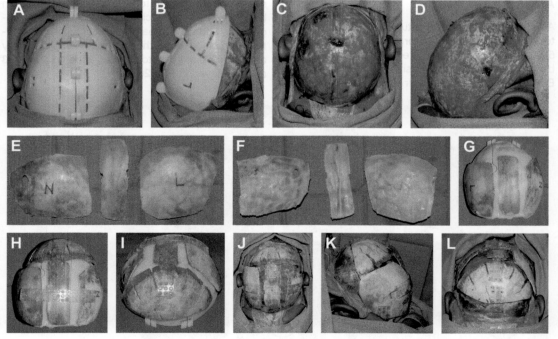

Fig. 25. Superior (*A*) and lateral (*B*) vies with cutting guide applied to cranial vault. Superior (*C*) and lateral (*D*) views with cranial vault removed. (*E, F*) External and internal views of the cranial vault segments. Note the thinning and perforations of the cranial vault. The bony segments are then switched to the contralateral side and applied with the sagittal suture segment to the bony repositioning (*G*). Superior (*H*) and poster (*I*) views of the fixated cranial vault on the positioning guide. Superior (*J*), lateral (*K*), and posterior (*L*) views of the reconstructed cranial complex applied to the patient's native cranium.

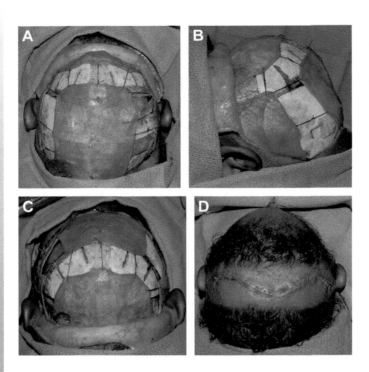

Fig. 26. Bird's-eye (*A*), lateral (*B*), and posterior (*C*) views demonstrating reapproximation of pericranial flaps and temporalis muscles. (*D*) A bird's-eye view after skin closure.

INTRODUCTION: NATURE OF THE PROBLEM— UNILATERAL LAMBDOID SYNOSTOSIS, POSTERIOR CRANIAL VAULT EXPANSION, AND REMODELING

Among the major cranial sutures, lambdoid synostosis is the least common form representing 3% to 5% of cases of single-suture synostosis.[31] It must be distinguished from positional plagiocephaly. Both produce an oblique or twisted head shape.

However, the latter stems from either intrauterine-pelvic constraint or secondary postnatal positional deformation such as repetitive sleep position and/or torticollis. Clinically this can be distinguished by clinical examination. Distinguishing and similar features of occipital asymmetry stemming from either posterior plagiocephaly and lambdoid synostosis are listed in **Table 3** and displayed in **Fig. 28**.[31–36]

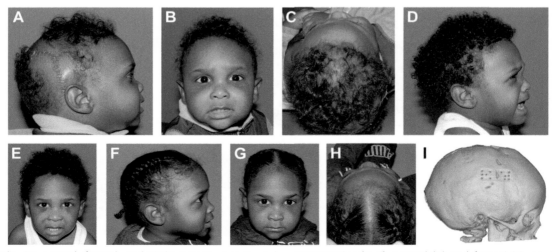

Fig. 27. Lateral, frontal, and Bird's-eye views at 2 weeks postoperative (*A–C*). Lateral (*D*) and frontal (*E*) views 1 year after surgery. Lateral, frontal, and bird's-eye views 2 years after surgery (*F–H*). Lateral view of CT taken 1 year after surgery (*I*).

Table 3	
Findings in posterior plagiocephaly and lambdoid synostosis	
Posterior Plagiocephaly	**Unilateral Lambdoid Synostosis**
Parallelogram from bird's-eye view	Trapezoid from bird's-eye view
Ipsilateral ear displaced anteriorly	Ipsilateral ear displaced posteriorly
Ipsilateral frontal bossing	Contralateral frontal bossing
Ipsilateral occipitoparietal flattening	Ipsilateral occipitoparietal flattening
No ipsilateral occipitoparietal bossing	Ipsilateral occipitoparietal bossing
Contralateral occipitoparietal bossing	Contralateral occipitoparietal bossing

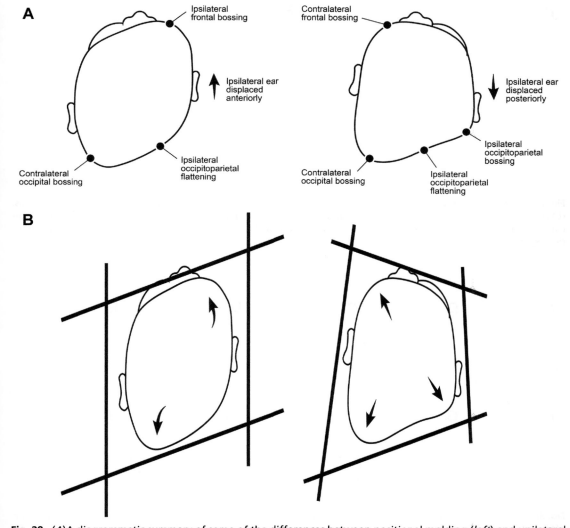

Fig. 28. (A)A diagrammatic summary of some of the differences between positional molding (*left*) and unilateral lambdoid synostosis (*right*). (*B*) Differences in head shape from bird's-eye view (*arrows* indicate directions of compensatory growth vectors). Positional molding produces parallelogram-shaped head (left). Unilateral lambdoid synostosis produces trapezoid shaped head (*right*). *(From* Huang MH, Gruss JS, Clarren SK, Mouradian WE, Cunningham ML, Roberts TS, Loeser JD, Cornell CJ. The differential diagnosis of posterior plagiocephaly: true lambdoid synostosis versus positional molding. Plast Reconstr Surg. 1996 Oct;98(5):765-74; discussion 775-6.).

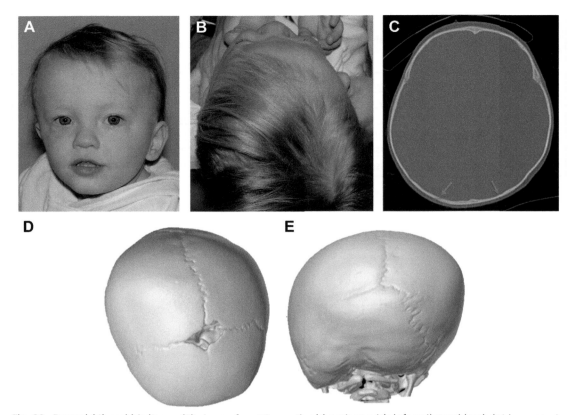

Fig. 29. Frontal (*A*) and bird's-eye (*B*) views of an 18-month-old patient with left unilateral lambdoid synostosis. (*C*) An axial view of CT of the same patient. (*Blue arrow* indicates patent right lambdoid suture; *red arrow* indicates fused left lambdoid suture). Bird's-eye (*D*) and posterior (*E*) 3D CT views demonstrating left unilateral lambdoid synostosis.

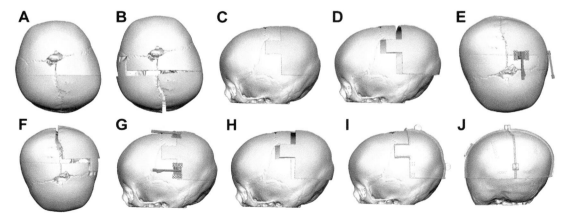

Fig. 30. (*A, B*) Bird's-eye views of the cranium before and after planned virtual expansion using a nondistraction plan and using bone grafting. (*C, D*) Lateral views of the cranium before and after planned virtual expansion. (*E, F*) Bird's-eye views of the cranium before and after planned virtual expansion using an approach using distraction osteogenesis. The STLS of distractors are imported into the virtual space, and distraction placement along with vector of movement can be evaluated. (*G, H*) Lateral views of the cranium before and after planned virtual expansion. (*I, J*) Bird's-eye and posterior views of virtually planned cutting guides used to replicate craniotomies in surgery.

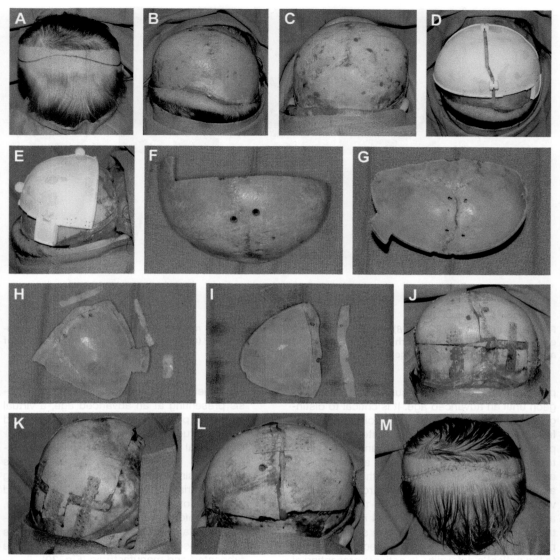

Fig. 31. Bird's-eye view of the patient in a prone position before incision (*A*). Bird's-eye (*B*) and posterior (*C*) views after reflection of pericranial flaps and temporalis muscles demonstrating left lambdoid synostosis. Bird's-eye (*D*) and lateral view (*E*) of the cutting guide applied to the cranial vault. The craniotomy segment is taken to the back table for planned osteotomies. (*F*) External view. (*G*) Internal view. Split-thickness bone grafts are harvested, and fixation is applied along with the desired plan (*H*, *I*). Bird's-eye (*J*), lateral (*K*), and posterior (*L*) views of the reconstructed cranial vault. Bird's-eye view after skin closure after reconstruction (*M*).

Similar to all cases of single suture craniosynostosis, the authors prefer an individualized approach to cranial vault expansion and remodeling for lambdoid synostosis with the goals of

1. Relieving the presence or the risk of raised intracranial pressure
2. Establishing normal cranial morphology and form
3. Establishing normal cephalic indices consistent with age-matched anthropometric norms

After clinical evaluation (**Fig. 29**A, B), radiographic confirmation of lambdoid synostosis in the form of a CT is imperative before considering a surgical procedure (**Fig. 29**C, E).

Indications/Contraindications

Lambdoid synostosis is rare and accounts for the least prevalent form of single suture synostosis. It is commonly misdiagnosed as posterior positional plagiocephaly, and patients often will not

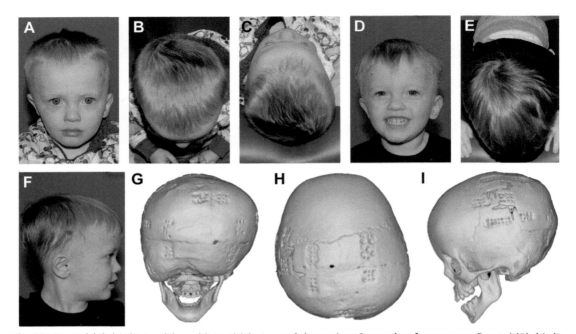

Fig. 32. Frontal (*A*), bird's-eye (*B*), and lateral (*C*) views of the patient 3 months after surgery. Frontal (*D*), bird's-eye (*E*), and lateral (*F*) views of the patient 1 year after surgery. Posterior (*G*), bird's-eye (*H*), and lateral (*I*) views of a 3D CT taken 1 year after surgery.

present to the craniofacial surgeon or neurosurgeon until an advanced age. It is critical to distinguish isolated unilateral lambdoid synostosis from occipital asymmetry from posterior plagiocephaly. In patients diagnosed with lambdoid synostosis at less than 5 months of age, an endoscopic assisted procedure with cranial orthosis is offered as an option in addition to standard open cranial vault corrective techniques. After this timeframe and before approximately 18 to 24 months of life, the authors will commonly offer a switch cranioplasty. However, the surgical procedure is tailored to the patient's deformity. In patients presenting at a later age (greater than 18–24 months of age), and depending on the morphology and thickness of the cranial vault, craniotomy with distraction osteogenesis is considered. However, the authors' preference is often for bilateral expansion and advancement of the posterior cranial vault with split-thickness bone grafting of full-thickness calvarial defects.

TECHNIQUE/PROCEDURE FOR LAMBDOID SUTURE CRANIOSYNOSTOSIS
Cranial Vault Remodeling

Preoperative planning

- Preoperative planning for open CVR for lambdoid synostosis is similar to that for sagittal suture synostosis.

- For patients with unilateral lambdoid synostosis presenting at an advanced age, a virtual computer planning session is carried out and a reconstruction is simulated that will establish normal cranial vault morphology and dimensions. In an older patient, the authors will often simulate a nondistraction plan using split calvarial bone grafting (**Fig. 30**A–D), and a distraction plan (**Fig. 30**E–H) to compare, with a preference for a single-stage nondistraction plan with bone grafting. Regardless of the chosen plan, virtual cutting guides are fabricated and manufactured (**Fig. 30**I, J).
- Similar to other forms of craniosynostosis the patient and family meet for consultation and discussion with Craniofacial, Neurosurgery, dysmorphology, and social work teams. For patients experiencing any form of neurodevelopmental delay, the patient and family will meet with the neuropsychologist on the craniofacial team.

PREPARATION AND PATIENT POSITIONING

Patient preparation and positioning is similar to that described previously (**Fig. 31**A).

Surgical Approach

- Incision, subgaleal dissection, followed by release and reflection of pericranial and bilateral temporalis flaps is performed as previously described (**Fig. 31**B, C)

- To plan for placement of fixation or distractors, subpericranial dissection often has to be performed 3 to 4 cm below the lambdoid suture. Just below the torcula, the surgeon will often encounter large venous vessels.
  - Judicious use of bone wax and meticulous hemostasis is critical to prevent potential air embolus in this area.

Surgical Procedure

Step 1: once the cranial vault is exposed, cutting guides are applied to the calvarium and craniotomy lines are marked with a sterile pencil (**Fig. 31**D, E).

Step 2: the neurosurgery team then completes the craniotomies. The posterior cranial vault is taken to the back table (**Fig. 31**F, G).

Step 3: the posterior vault is split in accordance with the preoperative plan, and split-thickness calvarial grafts are harvested for both sides of the cranial vault (**Fig. 31**H, I).

Step 4: the bony segments are then transferred over to the patient and secured with PDLLA/PLLA resorbable fixation (**Fig. 31**J–L). Segments of split-thickness bone graft are used to fill all areas of exposed dura; these are secured in place by either resorbable fixation or resorbable 2-0 polydioxanone suture.

Step 5: the periosteum and temporalis muscles are suspended using 3-0 Vicryl sutures. The galea aponeurotica is then closed using 3-0 Vicryl sutures.

Step 9: skin closure is done with a running 4-0 Vicryl Rapide suture (**Fig. 31**M).

Immediate Postoperative Care

- Immediate postoperative care is similar to that described previously.

Intermediate and Long-Term Postoperative Care

- Intermediate and long-term care is similar to that described previously. The patient is again seen 2 and 6 weeks postoperatively followed by 3 months (**Fig. 32**A–C), then 1 year (**Fig. 32**D–F), and yearly thereafter until the patient's cranial growth has ceased (**Fig. 32**G–I).

Possible Complications and Management

- Similar to previously described modified pi-plasty and CVR procedures for sagittal craniosynostosis.

Current Controversies/Future Considerations

Protocols for timing, type, and extent of repair for sagittal and lambdoid synostosis vary by surgeon and center. Rather than strict protocols on the procedure being performed, the authors prefer and advocate for an approach that is customized to the patient and aimed at addressing their specific deformity and dysmorphology. Endoscopic approaches with helmet therapy are beneficial at a young age, and the authors will certainly offer these approaches to families and patients who meet criteria. These minimally invasive procedures are discussed elsewhere in this text.

SUMMARY

When choosing an open approach to cranial vault expansion and remodeling, the authors will consider a variety of procedures and individualize the treatment to the patient with the goal of optimizing neurodevelopmental delay, establishing normal head shape and morphology, limiting morbidity to the patient, and preventing any inhibition of future growth.

CLINICS CARE POINTS

- When evaluating a patient for isolated sagittal craniosynostosis, the patient will often demonstrate restricted growth perpendicular to the fused suture with associated bitemporal and biparietal narrowing and compensatory growth parallel to the involved suture, which manifests as frontal and occipital bossing.

- The goals of surgical correction of craniosynostosis are to
  - limit external brain compression from the cranial vault
  - improve head shape and aesthetics to ideal established norms
  - promote normal craniofacial growth and neurodevelopment

- The choice of reconstructive technique for isolated sagittal suture craniosynostosis mostly depends on age of the patient and extent of the deformity.

- Careful attention to patient preparation and positioning is a critical to reducing patient comorbidity during the operation.

- Performing the modified pi-plasty in the suprapericranial/subgaleal plane reduces blood loss.

- Meticulous hemostasis during subgaleal dissection will minimize blood loss during the procedure.
- Cranial segments should be passive and nonoverlapping before closure.
- Given the rapid growth of the patient and cranial vault at this age, when using virtual planning, ideally the CT is taken within 4 weeks of the procedure to maximize the fit of the surgical cutting guides and templates.
- the neurosurgery team is performing the remainder of the craniotomies, the craniofacial team can reduce surgical time by using positioning guides and begin to reconstruct and fixate the cranial vault on the back table.
- The differentiation and diagnosis of unilateral lambdoid synostosis and posterior position plagiocephaly is based on the clinical examination. CT can confirm but should not be done unless the clinical examination suggests lambdoid synostosis.
- For patients who present with the diagnosis of unilateral lambdoid synostosis at a later age, nondistraction and distraction plans should be considered. Age of the patient, extent of the deformity, and virtual planning workup are key factors when considering either option. If equivocal in results, a nondistraction plan is preferred.

REFERENCES

1. Persing JA, Jane JA, Shaffrey M. Virchow and the pathogenesis of craniosynostosis: a translation of his original work. Plast Reconstr Surg 1989;83:738–42.
2. Delashaw JB, Persing JA, Broaddus WC, et al. Cranial vault growth in craniosynostosis. J Neurosurg 1989;70:159–65.
3. Lajeunie E, Le Merrer M, Bonaiti-Pellie C, et al. Genetic study of scaphocephaly. Am J Med Genet 1996;62:282–5.
4. Cohen MM Jr. Sutural biology and the correlates of craniosynostosis. Am J Med Genet 1993;47:581–616.
5. Hunter AG, Rudd NL. Craniosynostosis. I. Sagittal synostosis: its genetics and associated clinical findings in 214 patients who lacked involvement of the coronal suture(s). Teratology 1976;14:185–93.
6. Vollmer DG, Jane JA, Park TS, et al. Variants of sagittal synostosis: strategies for surgical correction. J Neurosurg 1984;61:557–62.
7. Roth DA, Bradley JP, Levine JP, et al. Studies in cranial suture biology: part II. Role of the dura in cranial suture fusion. Plast Reconstr Surg 1996;97:693–9.
8. Thompson DN, Harkness W, Jones B, et al. Subdural intracranial pressure monitoring in craniosynostosis: its role in surgical management. Childs Nerv Syst 1995;11:269–75.
9. Kapp-Simon KA, Speltz ML, Cunningham ML, et al. Neurodevelopment of children with single suture craniosynostosis: a review. Childs Nerv Syst 2007;23:269–81.
10. Anderson FM, Geiger L. Craniosynostosis: a survey of 204 cases. J Neurosurg 1965;22:229–40.
11. Duan M, Skoch J, Pan BS, et al. Neuro-ophthalmological manifestations of craniosynostosis: current perspectives. Eye Brain 2021;13:29–40.
12. Lannelongue M. De la craniectomie dans la microcéphalie. Compt Rend Seances Acad Sci 1890;50:1382–5.
13. Lane L. Pioneer craniectomy for relief of mental imbecility due to premature sutural closure and microcephalus. JAMA 1892;18:49–50.
14. Tessier P. [Total facial osteotomy. Crouzon's syndrome, Apert's syndrome: oxycephaly, scaphocephaly, turricephaly]. Ann Chir Plast 1967;12:273–86.
15. Tessier P, Guiot G, Rougerie J, et al. [Cranio-naso-orbito-facial osteotomies. Hypertelorism]. Ann Chir Plast 1967;12:103–18.
16. Rougerie J, Derome P, Anquez L. [Craniostenosis and cranio-facial dysmorphism. Principles of a new method of treatment and its results]. Neurochirurgie 1972;18:429–40.
17. Whitaker LA, Schut L, Kerr LP. Early surgery for isolated craniofacial dysostosis. Improvement and possible prevention of increasing deformity. Plast Reconstr Surg 1977;60:575–81.
18. Farkas LG, Posnick JC, Hreczko TM. Anthropometric growth study of the head. Cleft Palate Craniofac J 1992;29:303–8.
19. Christofides EA, Steinmann ME. A novel anthropometric chart for craniofacial surgery. J Craniofac Surg 2010;21:352–7.
20. Yen DW, Nguyen DC, Skolnick GB, et al. Evaluation of direct surgical remodeling of frontal bossing in patients with sagittal synostosis. J Craniofac Surg 2019;30:2350–4.
21. Hughes CD, Isaac KV, Hwang PF, et al. Modification of the melbourne method for total calvarial vault remodeling. Plast Reconstr Surg Glob Open 2018;6:e1848.
22. Khechoyan D, Schook C, Birgfeld CB, et al. Changes in frontal morphology after single-stage open posterior-middle vault expansion for sagittal craniosynostosis. Plast Reconstr Surg 2012;129:504–16.
23. Pattisapu JV, Gegg CA, Olavarria G, et al. Craniosynostosis: diagnosis and surgical management. Atlas Oral Maxillofac Surg Clin North Am 2010;18:77–91.
24. Jimenez DF, Barone CM. Endoscopic technique for sagittal synostosis. Childs Nerv Syst 2012;28:1333–9.

25. Monte TM, Denadai R, Raposo-Amaral CA, et al. Long-term morphologic changes on sagittal synostosis patients who underwent a modified Pi technique. J Craniofac Surg 2021;32:55–7.

26. Alperovich M, Runyan CM, Gabrick KS, et al. Long-term neurocognitive outcomes of spring-assisted surgery versus cranial vault remodeling for sagittal synostosis. Plast Reconstr Surg 2021;147:661–71.

27. Jones VM, Thomas SG, Siska R, et al. Spring-assisted surgery for treatment of sagittal craniosynostosis. J Craniofac Surg 2021;32:164–7.

28. Ruiz RL, Tiwana PS, Trent DC. Fronto-orbital advancement and anterior cranial vault reconstruction. In: Kademani D, Tiwana P, editors. Atlas of oral and maxillofacial surgery. New York: Saunders, an imprint of Elsevier, Inc; 2016.

29. Birgfeld CB, Dufton L, Naumann H, et al. Safety of open cranial vault surgery for single-suture craniosynostosis: a case for the multidisciplinary team. J Craniofac Surg 2015;26:2052–8.

30. McCarthy JG, Bradley JP, Stelnicki EJ, et al. Hung span method of scaphocephaly reconstruction in patients with elevated intracranial pressure. Plast Reconstr Surg 2002;109:2009–18.

31. Huang MH, Mouradian WE, Cohen SR, et al. The differential diagnosis of abnormal head shapes: separating craniosynostosis from positional deformities and normal variants. Cleft Palate Craniofac J 1998;35:204–11.

32. Birgfeld CB, Heike C. Distinguishing between lambdoid craniosynostosis and deformational plagiocephaly: a review of this paradigm shift in clinical decision-making and lesson for the future. Craniomaxillofac Trauma Reconstr 2020;13:248–52.

33. Ehret FW, Whelan MF, Ellenbogen RG, et al. Differential diagnosis of the trapezoid-shaped head. Cleft Palate Craniofac J 2004;41:13–9.

34. Ellenbogen RG, Gruss JS, Cunningham ML. Update on craniofacial surgery: the differential diagnosis of lambdoid synostosis/posterior plagiocephaly. Clin Neurosurg 2000;47:303–18.

35. Huang MH, Gruss JS, Clarren SK, et al. The differential diagnosis of posterior plagiocephaly: true lambdoid synostosis versus positional molding. Plast Reconstr Surg 1996;98:765–74 [discussion: 775-766].

36. Ploplys EA, Hopper RA, Muzaffar AR, et al. Comparison of computed tomographic imaging measurements with clinical findings in children with unilateral lambdoid synostosis. Plast Reconstr Surg 2009;123:300–9.

Management of Sagittal and Lambdoid Craniosynostosis
Minimally Invasive Approaches

Sameer Shakir, MD[1], Melissa Roy, MD[1], Amy Lee, MD,
Craig B. Birgfeld, MD*

KEYWORDS

- Endoscopic strip craniectomy • Spring-mediated cranioplasty • Minimally invasive
- Sagittal craniosynostosis • Lambdoid craniosynostosis • Cranial helmeting

KEY POINTS

- Less invasive techniques including endoscopic strip craniectomy with postoperative helmeting (ESC + PHT) and spring-mediated cranioplasty (SMC) offer at least comparable aesthetic outcomes to conventional open cranial vault remodeling with improved perioperative morbidity.
- In general, ESC and SMC modalities rely on underlying rapid brain growth and the viscoelastic nature of an infant's skull. These procedures ideally occur before 4 to 5 months of age.
- Although rare, elevated postoperative intracranial pressure requiring secondary open cranial vault remodeling has been reported to occur in individuals treated with ESC or SMC at an older age.
- Successful head shape correction in modern ESC interventions requires strict compliance with an extended period of postoperative helmeting.
- Cranial springs widen across a bone segment in an analogous manner to conventional distraction. They do not typically involve postoperative helmeting to normalize head shape but require a secondary surgery for hardware removal.

INTRODUCTION

Surgical techniques have evolved from simple strip craniectomies introduced by Lannelongue and Lane in the 1890s to open cranial vault remodeling (CVR) procedures popularized by Tessier in the 1970s with improving perioperative profiles. The resurgence of strip craniectomies began in the mid-1990s with advances in surgical technique and anesthesia coupled with the critical observation that earlier interventions benefitted from an easily molded skull. In their seminal work on endoscopically assisted strip craniectomy with postoperative helmeting (ESC + PHT) for the treatment of nonsyndromic sagittal craniosynostosis (SC),

Jimenez and Barone addressed 2 critiques of prevailing, open techniques: (1) most infants treated with a simple suturectomy around 2 to 3 months of age ultimately required subsequent CVR 6 months thereafter due to relapse in head shape dysmorphology; (2) open procedures were historically morbid, given the scalp incisions, blood loss, and lengthy operative times involved.[1] Their introduction of ESC + PHT in newborns and young infants not only offered decreased morbidity but also normalized head shape through a minimally invasive approach. Around the same time in Sweden, Claes Lauritzen introduced spring-mediated cranioplasty (SMC), which involved principles of gradual distraction based on torsion springs

University of Washington, Seattle Children's Hospital, 4800 Sand Point Way, Seattle, WA 98105, USA
[1] These authors contributed equally to the preparation of this article
* Corresponding author.
E-mail address: craig.birgfeld@seattlechildrens.org

Oral Maxillofacial Surg Clin N Am 34 (2022) 421–433
https://doi.org/10.1016/j.coms.2022.04.002
1042-3699/22/© 2022 Elsevier Inc. All rights reserved.

forces.[2] Thus began the era of minimally invasive approaches in the surgical correction of craniosynostosis. These techniques, which are used to treat a variety of craniosynostosis phenotypes, remain especially popular for the treatment of SC and unilambdoid craniosynostosis (ULS) across several high-volume centers.[3–8] The following article provides technical descriptions of these treatment modalities, a comparative literature review, and our institutional algorithms for the correction of SC and ULS.

CONSIDERATIONS FOR ENDOSCOPIC VERSUS OPEN TECHNIQUES

The universal goals of cranial vault surgery across all phenotypes include (1) optimizing cerebral blood flow via expansion of intracranial volume and (2) improving head shape. Reconstruction is an age-dependent approach with early diagnosis simplifying and directing operative management across all phenotypes.[9,10] Surgical timing carefully balances neurocognitive impact of disease, neurocognitive impact of interventions, and the potential need for revisional surgery. Despite the myriad of described operative techniques, these modalities involve either strip craniectomies or cranial vault remodeling. The prevailing controversy in operative management of nonsyndromic craniosynostosis remains comparative outcomes following less invasive strip craniectomies that use either SMC and/or PHT to help direct growth versus conventional, open CVR. Existing literature demonstrates less invasive techniques to offer comparable aesthetic outcomes to CVR with improved perioperative morbidity (ie, blood loss, transfusion rates, operative time, length of stay). In general, less invasive techniques including ESC and SMC rely on underlying rapid brain growth and the viscoelastic nature of an infant's skull. These procedures ideally occur before 4 to 5 months of age. Proponents of endoscopic suturectomy argue that suture release at an earlier age may account for improved outcomes related to subsequent craniofacial growth.[11,12] Contrastingly, open cranial vault remodeling procedures including frontoorbital advancement, posterior vault remodeling, and whole vault cranioplasty ideally occur between 6 and 12 months of age when (1) the brain's rapid growth provides an internal molding force postoperatively, (2) maturing yet malleable cranial bones allow for hardware fixation and reshaping, and (3) anesthetic risks are decreased. Beyond 18 months of age, CVR interventions may lead to persistent bony defects in an age-dependent manner presumably due to a less osteogenic dura mater.[13]

SAGITTAL CRANIOSYNOSTOSIS
Overview

Premature fusion of the sagittal suture leads to predictable cranial dysmorphology in the form of suture ridging, parietotemporal narrowing, and compensatory frontal bossing and occipital bulleting culminating in a decreased cephalic index $\left(\frac{biparietal\ diameter}{fronto-occipital\ diameter}x\ 100\right)$. Of the various craniosynostoses phenotypes, SC perhaps represents the greatest disparity in consensus management.[14] Proponents of open CVR argue this type of intervention alone normalizes multidimensional scaphocephaly in a single stage. Specifically, CVR techniques aim to expand regions of the skull inherently restricted by an overlying fused sagittal suture while reducing regions of the skull affected by compensatory growth.[15] Proponents of less invasive endoscopic strip craniectomies argue these techniques offer a comparable cranial expansion resulting from a rapidly expanding brain, decrease perioperative morbidity, and halt progressive deformity that may otherwise require more extensive remodeling.[1,16,17]

Endoscopic Strip Craniectomy with Postoperative Helmeting

In 1998, David Jimenez and Constance Barone reintroduced strip craniectomy for the treatment of SC with 2 major additions: (1) the use of endoscopes to minimize incisions and soft tissue dissection and (2) postoperative helmet therapy to redirect cranial growth into a more normocephalic shape.[1] Their surgical approach emphasized (1) small incisions, (2) endoscopic visualization of the surgical field, (3) suturectomy of the synostotic suture, and, perhaps most importantly, (4) the use of postoperative cranial molding therapy using customized helmets. Although existing literature fails to demonstrate any consistent differences in head shape with varying craniectomy widths or osteotomy patterns, several techniques have emerged.[18,19] Ridgway and colleagues[9] recommended removing a 1 cm strip of bone without barrel stave osteotomies. In contrast, Baker and colleagues[8,20] recommended removing a width of bone that inversely correlates with patient age, whereas the Synostosis Research Group reported a direct correlation between change in cephalic index (CI) and craniectomy width in patients undergoing strip craniectomy.

Jimenez's ESC + PHT procedure begins with two ~2 cm transverse incisions 2 cm posterior to the anterior fontanelle and immediately anterior to the lambda, centered on the sagittal suture **(Fig. 1)**. Following subgaleal dissection, extradural

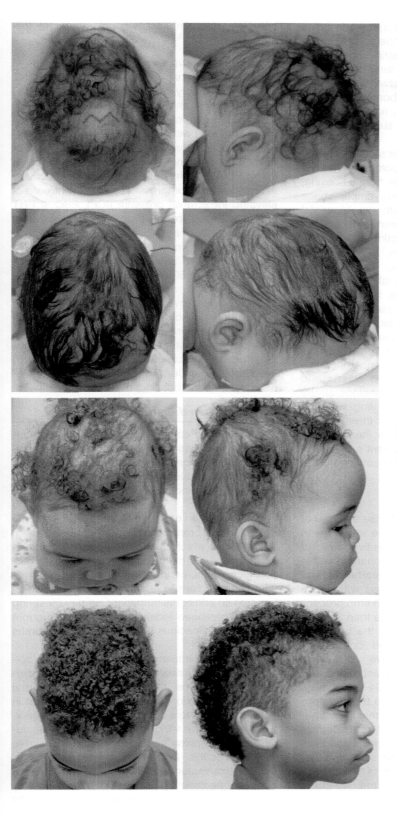

Fig. 1. Sagittal craniosynostosis. A 4-month-old man with classic scaphocephalic head shape and CI 65.8%. Note the operative marking involving two 2 cm zigzag incisions over the lambda and 2 cm posterior to the anterior fontanelle (*top*). Immediate postoperative result with closure of incisions using resorbable suture (*upper*). Three months postoperatively, note the improved frontooccipital diameter and biparietal widening with CI 72.1% (*lower*). Seven years postoperatively, he has maintained his head shape correction (*bottom*).

dissection occurs through parasagittal burr holes to minimize injury or tearing of the sagittal sinus. Bone scissors complete the strip craniectomy and are used to barrel stave the temporal and parietal bones to achieve transverse biparietal widening. The strip craniectomy bone is then delivered through the scalp incision, morselized, and orthotopically placed over the suturectomy site (**Figs. 2** and **3**).

Helmeting therapy corrects the scaphocephalic phenotype by applying gentle compression over areas of compensatory growth (ie, frontal bossing, occipital bulleting) and providing ample space over areas of restricted growth (ie, biparietal bones). The investigators recommended a 12-month helmeting protocol consisting of 3 helmets during 3 postoperative phases.[1] Phase 1 (ie, normalization) occurs during the first 2 months and aims to correct scaphocephaly. Phase 2 (ie, overcorrection) occurred for the next 4 months and aimed to overcorrect the head shape into a brachycephalic range. Phase 3 (ie, maintenance) occurs during the second half of the first postoperative year and aims to maintain normocephaly. Today, helmeting begins as early as postoperative day 5 following resolution of scalp edema and must be worn for 10 to 12 months postoperatively (or until the first birthday), correlating with the period of rapid brain growth. Two or three helmets may be necessary for complete head shape correction depending on the patient's age. Ultimately, head shape changes may continue up to 4 years postoperatively.[21]

Perioperative outcomes

In Jimenez and Barone's original case series, 3 of 4 patients remained transfusion free with a mean blood loss of 54 mL and operative time of 1.7 hours.[1] Most patients were discharged within 24 hours. These perioperative parameters and cost-savings significantly contrasted with those of open vault surgery and prior open strip procedures.[1] In an updated series of more than 850 patients undergoing ESC + PHT for the treatment of craniosynostosis, Jimenez and colleagues[8] report comparable perioperative outcomes (mean operative time [42–72 minutes], blood loss [10–32 mL], and length of stay [1.04–1.13 days]). Proctor and colleagues' experience treating nonsyndromic SC with ESC + PHT further substantiates these data.[9] In a 56-patient retrospective review, the investigators report a mean operative time of 45.3 minutes, transfusion rate of 3.6%, length of stay 1.39 days, and length of helmet therapy 7.47 months.[9] Throughout the literature, ESC + PHT interventions demonstrate a low incidence of perioperative blood transfusion, a short operative duration and hospital stay, and low morbidity.[1,8,9,21–23]

Morphometric outcomes

Aesthetic head shape outcomes in ESC + PHT compare favorably with conventional, open CVR in both short- and long-term follow-up.[17,23–25] Jimenez and Barone's 2004 review of 139 patients with SC treated with ESC + PHT reported a postoperative CI greater than 75% at a mean length of follow-up of 39 months in most of the patients (87%).[23] Although both techniques effectively relieve cerebral compression and prevent/correct elevated intracranial pressure (ICP), ESC + PHT is hypothesized to halt progressive cranial dysmorphology at an earlier age and perhaps reduce the necessity for more extensive remodeling.[8,9,17] Moreover, Shillito and colleagues'[26] review published in 1968 of 500+ patients with craniosynostosis suggested age of surgery to inversely correlate to improved head shape following strip craniectomy based on the cranial index and head circumference percentile. Nevertheless, existing literature demonstrates equivalent comparative head shape outcomes based on cephalic index, head circumference, and cephalometric (ie, euryonal height, frontal bossing) measures.[25,27]

Spring-Mediated Cranioplasty

In the 1980s, Persing and colleagues[28] demonstrated in rabbits that springs could enhance growth when placed across a craniectomy defect. Lauritzen subsequently published a case report on the use of expanding torsion springs to correct scaphocephaly.[29] The described procedure involved insertion of springs across a suturectomy site to slowly promote parietotemporal widening. The springs, which push apart 2 bony segments in an analogous manner to conventional distraction techniques, cannot be manipulated nor their vectors altered once placed. The technique, which requires an additional outpatient surgery for spring removal, has been widely adopted and is thought to be most efficacious if applied before 6 months of age.[3,6,7,10,30–32]

On the recommendation of Sood and colleagues,[33] preoperative helmeting may be considered at the time of initial evaluation at the surgeon's discretion until operative intervention in subjects with severe or worsening scaphocephaly. SMC may involve various patient positions (ie, supine, prone, "sphinx"), scalp incisions (ie, Chevron, "S", endoscopic access, long perpendicular to midline), craniectomy patterns (ie, sagittal suturectomy vs parasagittal craniectomy), craniectomy widths (ie, 1–4 cm), and spring designs (ie, "U" vs omega).[3,7,31,32,34,35] The investigators provide a

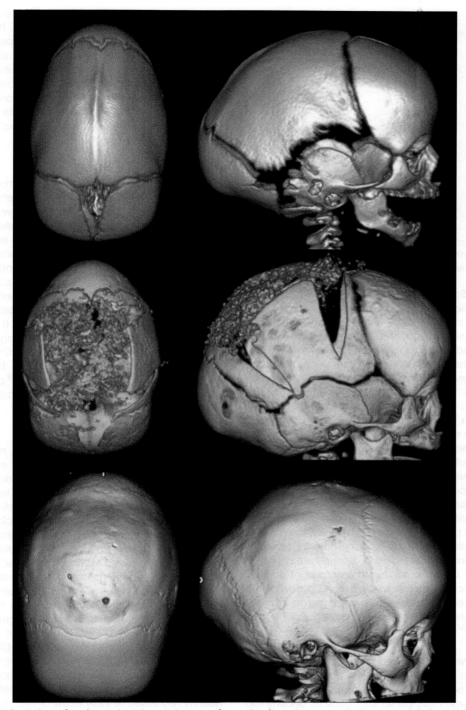

Fig. 2. CT depiction of endoscopic strip craniectomy for sagittal craniosynostosis. Preoperative depiction consisting of biparietal narrowing, occipital bulleting, and mild frontal bossing (*top*). Immediate postoperative imaging notable for wide strip craniectomy, parietotemporal barrel stave osteotomies, and orthotopic replacement of morselized bone (*middle*). Two-year postoperative CT imaging reveals a durable head shape correction with appropriate biparietal widening, increased posterior cranial height, and no full-thickness bony defects (*bottom*).

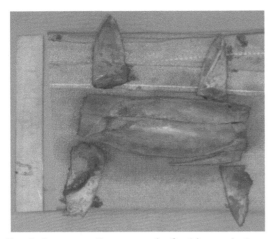

Fig. 3. Intraoperative removal of wide craniectomy bone with barrel parietotemporal barrel stave osteotomies.

multimedia demonstration of alternative operative approaches for SMC for SC.[36] Endoscopic visualization of the dura may be unnecessary, although it can be performed if the access incisions do not provide adequate visualization. Unlike most ESC interventions, SMC does not use parietotemporal barrel-stave osteotomies. Spring variables including gauge, length, and curvature may be altered to affect resultant spring force and expansile width.[34] Two to three springs may be inserted along the strip craniectomy segment with their footplates secured into bony notches. Out-of-plane bending of the springs allows for uniform force distribution without tenting of the overlying skin. Rodgers and colleagues[3] recommended an immediate 1 cm expansion on either side of the craniectomy defect that may be achieved by altering the spring variables previously discussed. Finally, the morselized craniectomy bone is orthotopically replaced and the incisions are closed. Springs are generally removed during a subsequent outpatient surgery 3 to 5 months afterward. A subgroup of patients may undergo postoperative helmeting to address severe saddling, occipital bossing, or frontal bossing.[37,38]

Perioperative outcomes

Similar to ESC + PHT, patients undergoing SMC benefit from improved perioperative and morbidity profiles when compared with patients undergoing conventional, open CVR. In their reporting of 225 patients undergoing SMC or CVR for the treatment of SC, Runyan and colleagues[6] reported significantly improved pooled perioperative outcomes (ie, mean blood loss, mean transfusion volume, operative time, and length of stay) across spring insertion and removal when compared with the CVR cohort.

In addition, Patel and colleagues[39] documented similarly rare perioperative outcomes (ie,. hemodynamic instability and neurologic decompensation) necessitating intensive care across patients undergoing SMC or CVR. In the quantitative analysis of 100 consecutive cases, The Great Ormond Street Hospital reported an overall complication rate of 9% with no mortalities, reoperation rate of 4%, and major complication rate of 1% related to iatrogenic injury of a parasagittal vein.[3]

Morphometric outcomes

SMC offers a durable head shape correction as determined by cephalic index. Lauritzen's initial report of patients with SC who underwent SMC included 35 patients between the ages of 2.5 and 8 months with mean spring removal occurring 7 months postoperatively.[32] Preoperative CI improved from 67% to 74% at the 6 months postoperative timepoint, and postoperative complications were limited to spring dislodgement (n = 3/35). Rodgers and colleagues reported a CI improvement from 68% to 72% at the 6 months timepoint, whereas Shakir and colleagues reported an improvement from 69% to 76% at the 5-year postoperative timepoint.[3,7] At 12 years postoperatively, Runyan and colleagues[6] provided the longest reported follow-up with improvement in CI from 70.7% to 75.7%.

Comparative outcomes

When compared with conventional CVR, minimally invasive techniques such as ESC + PHT and SMC provide notable improvements in perioperative morbidity and may be performed at an earlier age.[7,23–25,27] The durability of comparative head shape correction, however, remains unclear. In a 2018 comparison of patients undergoing ESC + PHT versus CVR for the correction of SC, Isaac and colleagues[27] reported comparably diminished head circumferences and cephalic indices at the 3-year postoperative timepoint. Runyan and colleagues'[6] long-term experience with SMC for the treatment of SC demonstrated a gradual increase in CI over 12 years (70.7% to 75.6%), whereas the CVR cohort demonstrated CI regression over 6 years (73.1% to 73.0%). van Veelen and colleagues'[35] series reported an increase in postoperative CI from 67% to 75% that subsequently regressed to 72% at the 5-year timepoint.

Direct comparison between minimally invasive techniques remains limited. Interestingly, the Pediatric Craniofacial Surgery Perioperative Registry concluded that ESC and SMC interventions resulted in similar transfusion-free hospital courses, but patients undergoing SMC had longer intensive care unit (ICU) and hospital lengths of

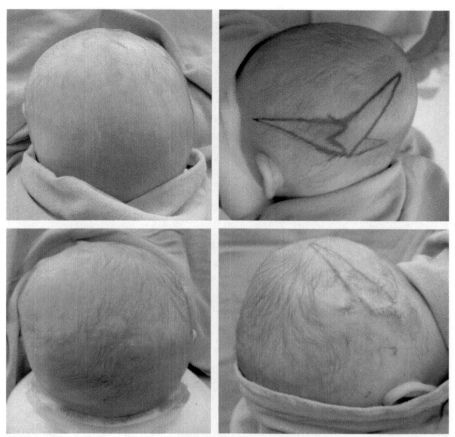

Fig. 4. Intraoperative depiction of unilambdoid craniosynostosis. Note the zigzag incision over the synostotic left lambdoid suture and planned barrel stave osteotomies (*purple*) (*upper right*). The incision is closed with absorbable suture (*bottom right*).

stay.[40] Although successful head shape correction in ESC procedures hinges on compliance with helmeting therapy, SMC interventions all require a secondary operative procedure for spring removal, irrespective of potential hardware failure that may prompt additional operative interventions. As the rate of preoperative and postoperative elevated ICP remains exceedingly low in the nonsyndromic, single-suture patient population, both treatment modalities demonstrate similar postoperative rates of elevated ICP requiring secondary CVR. Moreover, existing literature suggests most patients who develop postoperative elevated ICP or require secondary CVR for functional or aesthetic concerns underwent initial ESC or SMC beyond 6 months of age.[3,6,7,9,35]

UNILAMBDOID CRANIOSYNOSTOSIS
Overview

ULS poses diagnostic challenges due to a phenotype that resembles deformational plagiocephaly.[41,42] Key features include trapezoidal head shape, ipsilateral skull base tilt of the affected side, ipsilateral mastoid bulge, ipsilateral occipital flattening, and pronounced hemifacial deficiency (**Figs. 4** and **5**).[43,44] Other associated dysmorphic features relate to the cranial base deformities originating from the affected suture causing growth restriction and include an enlarged contralateral middle cranial fossa, a pronounced petrous ridge angle, and posterior fossa deviation toward the affected side.[45,46] Early diagnosis of ULS remains crucial to allow for timely assessment and consideration for age-dependent minimally invasive approaches. Minimally invasive modalities for the treatment of ULS invariably provide shorter anesthesia time, decreased blood loss, decreased length of stay, and comparable outcomes when compared with conventional, open CVR.[47]

Endoscopic Strip Craniectomy with Postoperative Helmeting

After induction of general anesthesia, the patient is placed in a prone position on a horseshoe

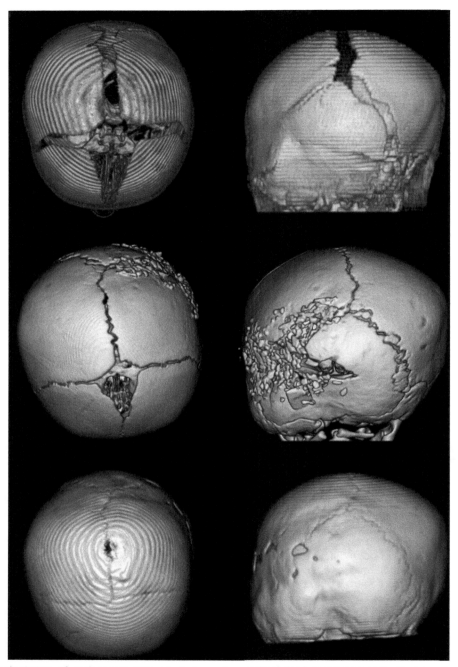

Fig. 5. CT depiction of endoscopic strip craniectomy for unilambdoid craniosynostosis. Preoperative imaging demonstrates a partially fused left lambdoid suture with ipsilateral skull base tilt and mastoid bulge (*top*). Immediate postoperative imaging notable for left lambdoid suturectomy and barrel stave osteotomies with orthotopic replacement of morselized bone (*middle*). Two-year postoperative imaging reveals improved cranial contour without full-thickness bony defects (*bottom*).

headrest. A 3 cm zigzag incision is marked on the inferior most aspect of the fused lambdoid suture (see **Fig. 4**). The planned craniectomy is marked, which includes the suturectomy site and barrel stave osteotomies extending just beneath the occiput, along the temporal bone, and above the squamosal bone. After the subgaleal plane is accessed, the scalp is elevated to expose the

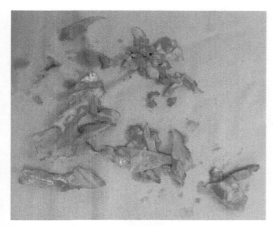

Fig. 6. Morselized bone graft. Bone graft is orthotopically placed along the suturectomy and osteotomy sites.

occiput, the fused lambdoid suture, and the ipsilateral temporal bone where barrel stave osteotomies will be made. Using a craniotomy burr, the anterior cranial space is accessed and the proposed craniectomy of the fused suture and barrel stave osteotomies are marked onto the scalp. Burr holes at the anterior aspect of the fused lambdoid suture are drilled and then widened using a Kerrison punch. The osteotomy between the burr holes is completed to allow for complete epidural space access and dissection. The endoscope is then used to visualize the epidural space and complete the epidural dissection. The dura is then protected with malleable retractors, and bone scissors are used to sharply excise the fused suture and create barrel stave osteotomies. Additional barrel stave osteotomies are made along the mastoid bulge. Morselized bone graft is placed into the skull defects (**Figs. 5** and **6**). The scalp is then reflected and closed in layers including the galea and skin. **Fig. 7** illustrates long-term postoperative outcomes.

Zubovic and colleagues[46] compared preoperative and 1-year postoperative computed tomography (CT) imaging of patients with ULS who underwent CVR (n = 8) versus ESC + PHT (n = 4). Anthropometric measurements were performed including posterior fossa deflection angle, petrous ridge angle, mastoid cant angle, and vertical and anterior-posterior displacement of the external acoustic meatus. Postoperative comparisons of the CVR and ESC cohorts did not show any statistically significant differences. Both cohorts demonstrated comparably reduced posterior cranial vault asymmetries with persistent cranial base and posterior cranial vault asymmetries and overall equivalent postoperative

outcomes. Rattani and colleagues[5] similarly reviewed a series of patients with ULS who underwent either CVR or ESC + PHT. Perioperative outcomes included operative time (mean 3 hours vs 1 hour [CVR vs ESC]) and estimated blood loss (mean 210 mL vs 25 mL [CVR vs ESC]). The investigators again noted comparable correction of occipital asymmetries in both cohorts without significant differences in head circumferences. Consequently, the investigators advocate for ESC + PHT for patients who present with ULS before 3 months of age.

Spring-Mediated Cranioplasty

SMC allows for progressive cranial vault reshaping via bony distraction and soft tissue expansion, likely contributing to lower rates of wound complications and relapse.[32,48,49] Arnaud and colleagues[48] first reported on the use of translambdoid springs through patent lambdoid sutures. In patients younger than 6 months (n = 19) with brachycephaly, the technique resulted in progressive increases in the posterior skull volume.[47] Similarly, the Rotterdam group highlighted their SMC experience in posterior vault expansion for multisuture craniosynostosis.[49] In comparing SMC (n = 15) with conventional posterior vault expansion using internal distractors (n = 16), the investigators demonstrate SMC to correlate with a larger increase in skull circumference and frontooccipital length. They concluded that SMC was a useful alternative to CVR in young children. Mittermiller and colleagues[4] subsequently published a retrospective review of patients with ULS undergoing SMC at mean age of 9.4 months. The investigators' results demonstrated improved aesthetic appearances, improvements in skull base symmetry, decreased operative times (mean 61 minutes), and decreased lengths of stay (mean 1.9 days).

Comparative Outcomes

ULS remains a rare entity, as it accounts for only 2% of all craniosynostoses.[43] The literature reflects the rarity of the diagnosis, as very few studies explore minimally invasive approaches and only include single institution experiences with limited sample sizes and short-term follow-up.[50] Nevertheless, there is evidence that ESC provides similar outcomes to conventional open CVR (ie, switch cranioplasty).[5,46] Endoscopic procedures carry less perioperative risk with comparable morphometric outcomes to CVR modalities while restoring nonsynostotic physiology sooner and directing growth by virtue of a molding helmet during the period of rapid brain growth.[5]

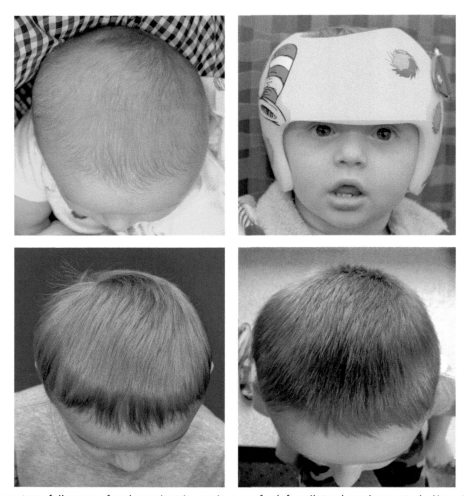

Fig. 7. Long-term follow-up of endoscopic strip craniectomy for left unilateral craniosynostosis. Note the ipsilateral mastoid bulge and ipsilateral occipital flattening (*upper left*). Patient presents during the early postoperative period with a cranial orthosis used to manipulate skull growth (*upper right*). He is seen 2 years postoperatively (*bottom left*) and 4 years postoperatively with a durable head shape correction (*bottom right*).

Independent of treatment modality, however, persistent cranial base and posterior vault asymmetries are associated with both techniques.[45,46] Specifically, persistent retrodisplacement of the contralateral middle cranial fossa and twisting of the posterior fossa toward the affected suture have been noted postoperatively after CVR. These constant cranial base deformities potentially have a long-term impact on facial growth that has yet to be determined.[45]

SMC for the correction of ULS remains poorly studied, although the technique has been successfully used for posterior vault expansion in the context of multisuture craniosynostosis.[48,49] Successful outcomes have been reported with some improvement in cranial base asymmetries, general cranial appearance, and no reported perioperative complications.[4] Its surgical role has been described as a minimally invasive approach that may be offered to children up to 18 months of age with reportedly satisfactory outcomes. Further studies with more detailed anthropometric analyses and long-term data would be necessary to better support SMC interventions for the management of ULS.

SEATTLE CHILDREN'S HOSPITAL TREATMENT PATHWAY

Patients presenting at or before 4 months of age are potential candidates for endoscopic craniectomy with postoperative helmeting or open CVR depending on parental preference. Both surgical techniques are described to the parents as well as expectations for recovery and planned follow-up visits. Transfusion rates are discussed (100%

for open vs 5% for endoscopic on most recent review). Scar expectations and duration of helmet therapy, if indicated, are described, and the location of the nearest orthotist to the patients' residence is located to estimate travel time. The parents are then left to decide.

Open treatment of SC involves a modified Pi procedure performed at 4 to 6 months of age, whereas open treatment of ULS involves a switch cranioplasty performed at 6 to 9 months of age. The authors do not currently perform SMC for the treatment of SC or ULS. Following surgery and extubation, patients undergo immediate CT imaging to rule out intracranial pathology only if an intraoperative event raises concern. Endoscopic patients are admitted to the general ward after recovery in the postanesthesia care unit. Open patients are admitted directly to the ICU. Prophylactic antibiotics are continued for a total of 24 hours postoperatively. Initial postoperative monitoring parameters encompass hemodynamic stability, pain control, neurologic examination, and oral intake. On postoperative day 1, patients who underwent open procedure undergo morning laboratory draws to evaluate for hemodynamic instability and transfer to the general ward. Scheduled laboratory draws are not performed on endoscopic patients unless clinically indicated. Most patients remain admitted between 1 and 3 days (average 1.5 days for endoscopic and 2.5 days for open). Specific discharge criteria include temperature less than 38°C for the last 24 hours, adequate oral pain control, tolerating enteral feeds, and decreasing facial edema.

Postoperative helmet therapy, which is integral to the postoperative pathway, takes place in collaboration with the orthotists at Seattle Children's Hospital or Hanger Clinic orthotists closer to home. A helmet is fitted on postoperative day 10 and delivered on postoperative day 14. It is then worn 23 hours a day for a period of 10 to 12 months with biweekly adjustments. The patient returns for an initial postoperative evaluation at 2 to 3 weeks for incision check and helmet fit assessment. The patient is then followed clinically by the surgeon every 4 to 6 weeks to monitor helmet molding with close collaboration between the craniofacial nurse and the orthotist in between.

CLINICS CARE POINTS

- The incidence of postoperative neurologic or hemodynamic deterioration is exceedingly low in patients with nonsyndromic craniosynostosis undergoing endoscopic strip craniectomy with postoperative helmeting or SMC, obviating postoperative intensive care.
- The decision to pursue endoscopic strip craniectomy versus open cranial vault remodeling often hinges on perceived compliance with postoperative helmeting.
- Out-of-plane bending of cranial springs allows for uniform force distribution without tenting of the overlying skin and mitigates soft tissue complications and concerns for hardware dislodgement.
- When performing SMC for SC, the risk of hardware failure requiring reoperation may be lessened when using 3 springs compared with 2.

REFERENCES

1. Jimenez DF, Barone CM. Endoscopic craniectomy for early surgical correction of sagittal craniosynostosis. J Neurosurg 1998;88(1):77–81.
2. Lauritzen C, Friede H, Elander A, et al. Dynamic cranioplasty for brachycephaly. Plast Reconstr Surg 1996;98(1):7–14 [discussion: 15-16].
3. Rodgers W, Glass GE, Schievano S, et al. Spring-assisted cranioplasty for the correction of nonsyndromic scaphocephaly: a quantitative analysis of 100 consecutive cases. Plast Reconstr Surg 2017;140(1):125–34.
4. Mittermiller PA, Rochlin DH, Menard RM. Endoscopic Spring-Mediated Distraction for Unilambdoid Craniosynostosis. J Craniofac Surg 2020;31(7):2097–100.
5. Rattani A, Riordan CP, Meara JG, et al. Comparative analysis of cranial vault remodeling versus endoscopic suturectomy in the treatment of unilateral lambdoid craniosynostosis. J Neurosurg Pediatr 2020;26(2):105–12.
6. Runyan CM, Gabrick KS, Park JG, et al. Long-term outcomes of spring-assisted surgery for sagittal craniosynostosis. Plast Reconstr Surg 2020;146(4):833–41.
7. Shakir S, Humphries LS, Kalmar CL, et al. Hope springs eternal: insights into the durability of springs to provide long-term correction of the scaphocephalic head shape. J Craniofac Surg 2020;31(7):2079–83.
8. Jimenez DF, Moon HS. Endoscopic approaches to craniosynostosis. Atlas Oral Maxillofac Surg Clin North Am 2022;30(1):63–73.
9. Ridgway EB, Berry-Candelario J, Grondin RT, et al. The management of sagittal synostosis using endoscopic suturectomy and postoperative helmet therapy. J Neurosurg Pediatr 2011;7(6):620–6.

10. Sun J, Ter Maaten NS, Mazzaferro DM, et al. Spring-mediated cranioplasty in sagittal synostosis: does age at placement affect expansion? J Craniofac Surg 2018;29(3):632–5.

11. Isaac KV, MacKinnon S, Dagi LR, et al. Nonsyndromic unilateral coronal synostosis: a comparison of fronto-orbital advancement and endoscopic suturectomy. Plast Reconstr Surg 2019;143(3):838–48.

12. Jimenez DF, Barone CM. Early treatment of anterior calvarial craniosynostosis using endoscopic-assisted minimally invasive techniques. Childs Nerv Syst 2007;23(12):1411–9.

13. Paige KT, Vega SJ, Kelly CP, et al. Age-dependent closure of bony defects after frontal orbital advancement. Plast Reconstr Surg 2006;118(4):977–84.

14. Doumit GD, Papay FA, Moores N, et al. Management of sagittal synostosis: a solution to equipoise. J Craniofac Surg 2014;25(4):1260–5.

15. Fearon JA. Evidence-based medicine: Craniosynostosis. Plast Reconstr Surg 2014;133(5):1261–75.

16. Gerety PA, Basta MN, Fischer JP, et al. Operative management of nonsyndromic sagittal synostosis: a head-to-head meta-analysis of outcomes comparing 3 techniques. J Craniofac Surg 2015; 26(4):1251–7.

17. Fearon JA, McLaughlin EB, Kolar JC. Sagittal craniosynostosis: surgical outcomes and long-term growth. Plast Reconstr Surg 2006;117(2):532–41.

18. Wood BC, Ahn ES, Wang JY, et al. Less is more: does the addition of barrel staves improve results in endoscopic strip craniectomy for sagittal craniosynostosis? J Neurosurg Pediatr 2017;20(1):86–90.

19. Dlouhy BJ, Nguyen DC, Patel KB, et al. Endoscope-assisted management of sagittal synostosis: wide vertex suturectomy and barrel stave osteotomies versus narrow vertex suturectomy. J Neurosurg Pediatr 2016;25(6):674–8.

20. Baker CM, Ravindra VM, Gociman B, et al. Management of sagittal synostosis in the Synostosis Research Group: baseline data and early outcomes. Neurosurg Focus 2021;50(4):E3.

21. Jimenez DF, Barone CM, Cartwright CC, et al. Early management of craniosynostosis using endoscopic-assisted strip craniectomies and cranial orthotic molding therapy. Pediatrics 2002;110(1 Pt 1): 97–104.

22. Barone CM, Jimenez DF. Endoscopic craniectomy for early correction of craniosynostosis. Plast Reconstr Surg 1999;104(7):1965–73 [discussion: 1974-1965].

23. Jimenez DF, Barone CM, McGee ME, et al. Endoscopy-assisted wide-vertex craniectomy, barrel stave osteotomies, and postoperative helmet molding therapy in the management of sagittal suture craniosynostosis. J Neurosurg 2004;100(5):407–17.

24. Guimaraes-Ferreira J, Gewalli F, David L, et al. Clinical outcome of the modified pi-plasty procedure for sagittal synostosis. J Craniofac Surg 2001;12(3): 218–24 [discussion: 225-216].

25. Heller JB, Heller MM, Knoll B, et al. Intracranial volume and cephalic index outcomes for total calvarial reconstruction among nonsyndromic sagittal synostosis patients. Plast Reconstr Surg 2008;121(1): 187–95.

26. Shillito J Jr, Matson DD. Craniosynostosis: a review of 519 surgical patients. Pediatrics 1968;41(4): 829–53.

27. Isaac KV, Meara JG, Proctor MR. Analysis of clinical outcomes for treatment of sagittal craniosynostosis: a comparison of endoscopic suturectomy and cranial vault remodeling. J Neurosurg Pediatr 2018; 22(5):467–74.

28. Persing JA, Babler WJ, Nagorsky MJ, et al. Skull expansion in experimental craniosynostosis. Plast Reconstr Surg 1986;78(5):594–603.

29. Lauritzen C, Sugawara Y, Kocabalkan O, et al. Spring mediated dynamic craniofacial reshaping. Scand J Plast Reconstr Surg Hand Surg 1998; 32(3):331–8.

30. Taylor JA, Maugans TA. Comparison of spring-mediated cranioplasty to minimally invasive strip craniectomy and barrel staving for early treatment of sagittal craniosynostosis. J Craniofac Surg 2011; 22(4):1225–9.

31. David LR, Plikaitis CM, Couture D, et al. Outcome analysis of our first 75 spring-assisted surgeries for scaphocephaly. J Craniofac Surg 2010;21(1):3–9.

32. Lauritzen CGK, Davis C, Ivarsson A, et al. The evolving role of springs in craniofacial surgery: the first 100 clinical cases. Plast Reconstr Surg 2008; 121(2):545–54.

33. Sood S, Rozzelle A, Shaqiri B, et al. Effect of molding helmet on head shape in nonsurgically treated sagittal craniosynostosis. J Neurosurg Pediatr 2011;7(6):627–32.

34. Shakir S, Humphries LS, Lanni MA, et al. What is the Role of Force in Correcting Scaphocephaly Through Spring-Mediated Cranial Vault Expansion for Sagittal Craniosynostosis? J Craniofac Surg 2021;32(8): 2615–20.

35. van Veelen MC, Kamst N, Touw C, et al. Minimally Invasive, Spring-Assisted Correction of Sagittal Suture Synostosis: Technique, Outcome, and Complications in 83 Cases. Plast Reconstr Surg 2018; 141(2):423–33.

36. Kalmar CL, Swanson JW, Shakir S, et al. Spring-mediated cranioplasty for sagittal craniosynostosis. Neurosurg Focus 2021;4:2–V6. https://doi.org/10.3171/2021.1.FOCVID2060. Available at:.

37. Marupudi NI, Sood S, Rozzelle A, et al. Effect of molding helmets on intracranial pressure and head shape in nonsurgically treated sagittal craniosynostosis patients. J Neurosurg Pediatr 2016;18(2): 207–12.

38. Swanson JW, Haas JA, Mitchell BT, et al. The Effects of Molding Helmet Therapy on Spring-Mediated Cranial Vault Remodeling for Sagittal Craniosynostosis. J Craniofac Surg 2016;27(6):1398–403.

39. Patel V, Shakir S, Yang R, et al. Perioperative Outcomes in the Treatment of Isolated Sagittal Synostosis: Cranial Vault Remodeling Versus Spring Mediated Cranioplasty. J Craniofac Surg 2020; 31(7):2106–11.

40. Lang SS, Meier PM, Paden WZ, et al. Spring-mediated cranioplasty versus endoscopic strip craniectomy for sagittal craniosynostosis. J Neurosurg Pediatr 2021;28(4):416–24.

41. Birgfeld CB, Heike C. Distinguishing between lambdoid craniosynostosis and deformational plagiocephaly: a review of this paradigm shift in clinical decision-making and lesson for the future. Craniomaxillofac Trauma Reconstr 2020;13(4):248–52.

42. Haas-Lude K, Wolff M, Will B, et al. Clinical and imaging findings in children with non-syndromic lambdoid synostosis. Eur J Pediatr 2014;173(4):435–40.

43. Borad V, Cordes EJ, Liljeberg KM, et al. Isolated Lambdoid Craniosynostosis. J Craniofac Surg 2019;30(8):2390–2.

44. Smartt JM Jr, Reid RR, Singh DJ, et al. True lambdoid craniosynostosis: long-term results of surgical and conservative therapy. Plast Reconstr Surg 2007;120(4):993–1003.

45. Elliott RM, Smartt JM Jr, Taylor JA, et al. Does conventional posterior vault remodeling alter endocranial morphology in patients with true lambdoid synostosis? J Craniofac Surg 2013;24(1):115–9.

46. Zubovic E, Woo AS, Skolnick GB, et al. Cranial Base and Posterior Cranial Vault Asymmetry After Open and Endoscopic Repair of Isolated Lambdoid Craniosynostosis. J Craniofac Surg 2015;26(5): 1568–73.

47. Proctor MR, Meara JG. A review of the management of single-suture craniosynostosis, past, present, and future. J Neurosurg Pediatr 2019;24(6):622–31.

48. Arnaud E, Marchac A, Jeblaoui Y, et al. Spring-assisted posterior skull expansion without osteotomies. Childs Nerv Syst 2012;28(9):1545–9.

49. de Jong T, van Veelen ML, Mathijssen IM. Spring-assisted posterior vault expansion in multisuture craniosynostosis. Childs Nerv Syst 2013;29(5):815–20.

50. Reardon T, Fiani B, Kosarchuk J, et al. Management of Lambdoid Craniosynostosis: A Comprehensive and Systematic Review. Pediatr Neurosurg 2022; 57(1):1–16.

Management of Minor Suture Craniosynostosis

Alisa O. Girard, MBS[a], Robin Yang, MD, DDS[a,b],*

KEYWORDS

• Minor suture craniosynostosis • Intracranial pathology • Scaphocephaly • Craniosynostosis

KEY POINTS

• Identification of minor suture craniosynostosis can vary in its presentation.
• Minor suture craniosynostosis is still a cause of intracranial pressure.
• Management and treatment should address the deformity as well as expansion.

BACKGROUND

Craniosynostosis describes a process that involves the fusion of one or more of the cranial sutures. It has an overall prevalence of 1 in 2500 live births.[1] During infancy, the infant calvarium grows to accommodate the expanding neural contents. The different bones of the skull are separated by narrow seams whereby most of the growth occurs. These seams of growth are termed cranial sutures. The topography of the infant skull can be depicted as geometric arches.[2] These cranial arches consist of both major and minor sutures. The sagittal arch consists of the sagittal and metopic major sutures as well as the frontonasal and ethmoid minor sutures. The sagittal and metopic sutures separate the paired frontal and parietal bones. The coronal arch consists of the paired coronal major sutures. At the cranial base, the coronal sutures divide into the frontosphenoidal (FS), sphenoethmoidal, and sphenosquamosal minor sutures. The coronal sutures separate the paired frontal and parietal bones laterally. The lambdoid major sutures separate the parietal bones posteriorly from a single occipital bone.[3] The lesser known squamosal arch joins the coronal and lambdoidal arches and contains the minor squamosal and parietomastoid sutures (**Fig. 1**).

TIMING OF SUTURE CLOSURE

The major sutures are reported to close later in adulthood. The exception is the metopic suture which can close as early as 3 months of age.[4] More recent studies also confirm that the squamosal sutures remain patent into adulthood.[5–7] Less is known about the minor sutures of the skull base as well as the synchondroses. Most are thought to close by the end of adolescence or correspond with the cessation of facial growth.[2] The increase in publications on the premature fusion of the minor sutures has resulted in more awareness as causes for physical differences in the infant calvarium. Much like major suture craniosynostosis, minor suture craniosynostosis can be associated neurologic complications which should be monitored or corrected.[8]

CLINICAL PRESENTATION

The aim of management of craniosynostosis should involve proper diagnosis, identification of other features that may suggest a syndromic process, and lastly the urgency of intervention. The most common presentation is a patient within their first year of life with an unusual shape of the head, forehead, and or orbit. Morphologic differences are usually classified as scaphocephaly/

a Department of Plastic and Reconstructive Surgery, Johns Hopkins University, Baltimore, MD, USA;
b Department of Plastic and Reconstructive Surgery, Johns Hopkins Hospital, 601 North Caroline Street, Baltimore, MD 21231, USA
* Corresponding author.
E-mail address: ryang14@jhmi.edu

Oral Maxillofacial Surg Clin N Am 34 (2022) 435–442
https://doi.org/10.1016/j.coms.2022.02.003

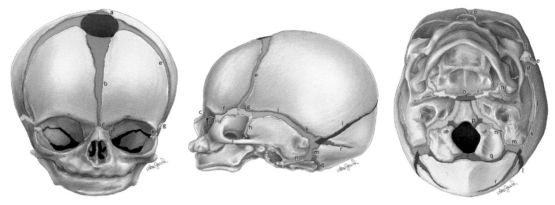

Fig. 1. Sutural arches of the neonatal skull in anterior (left), lateral (middle), and basal (right) views. Sagittal arch includes the sagittal (A), metopic (B), frontonasal (C), and frontoethmoidal D) sutures. Coronal arch includes the coronal (E), frontosphenoidal (F), sphenoparietal (G), sphenosquamous (H), and sphenopetrosal (I) sutures. The terminal suture of the anterior branch of the coronal arch (ethmoidal sphenoidal) is not shown. The squamosal arch includes the parieto squamous (J) and parietomastoid (K) sutures. The lambdoid arch consists of the lambdoid suture (L) and (M) and petro-occipital (N) synchondroses. The skull base sutures/synchondroses include the spheno-occipital (O), anterior intraoccipital (P), posterior intraoccipital (Q), and mendosal (R). (*Courtesy of* Alisa O. Girard, MBS, Baltimore, MD)

dolicocephaly, trigonocephaly, or anterior/posterior plagiocephaly. These head shapes are well documented and associated with the specific suture involvement (ie, sagittal craniosynostosis and scaphocephaly). The resulting calvarial differences largely comply with Virchow law, with restricted grown perpendicular to and compensatory growth at nonfused sutures parallel to the affected suture.

Recent literature indicates that isolated minor suture craniosynostosis is relatively infrequent.[9–11] In addition, the clinical presentation varied from scaphocephalic, plagiocephalic, and normal.[12,13] Most reported cases of minor suture involvement also involve craniosynostosis of the major sutures, which also dominate the morphologic calvarial shape.[2,8,12]

Suspicion of minor suture craniosynostosis should trigger practitioners to focus on any family history of unusual head shapes, prenatal exposures, and birth history. Clinical information should focus on functional consequences of potential multi-suture or syndromic craniosynostosis. Important clinical information should pertain to feeding, orbital protection, airway, and signs of elevated intra-cranial pressure (headaches, seizures, irritability, vomiting).

DIAGNOSTIC TESTING

Clinical diagnosis is often considered the gold standard for the diagnosis of craniosynostosis. When minor suture craniosynostosis is suspected, a computed tomography scan with three-

dimensional reconstruction is warranted. A CT will allow the evaluation of all sutures and patency. In addition, imaging of the brain will rule in or rule out any anatomic abnormalities such as hydrocephalous or chiari malformation (**Fig. 2**). In certain instances, an MRI with contrast or a venogram maybe indicated if there is a concern for abnormal venous drainage in the posterior fossa.[13]

SURGICAL INTERVENTION

The prevalence of elevated intra-cranial pressure in isolated single suture craniosynostosis is often reported to be less than 5%. In the syndromic or

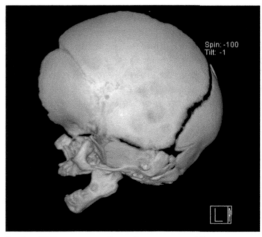

Fig. 2. CT Reconstruction of a patent with Aperts syndrome and bicoronal craniosynostosis.

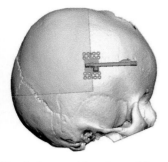
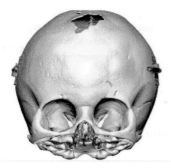
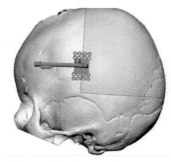

Fig. 3. 3-year-old patient with multisuture craniosynostosis, with both turricephaly and brachycephaly. Posterior cranial vault distraction to allow for expansion.

multi-suture patient, this number can be as high as 25%. Patients with signs of elevated intracranial pressure should receive more urgent intervention. In our institution, patients are evaluated by neuro-ophthalmology and started on Acetazolamide, if there is any sign of papilledema or elevated intra-cranial pressure. This will allow for a short-term decrease in intra-cranial pressure while they are prepared for surgical intervention.

The goals of intervention involve:

1. Expansion of the calvarium to decrease the intracranial pressure
2. Normalize head shape.

SYNDROMIC/BICORONAL CRANIOSYNOSTOSIS (BRACHYCEPHALY)

In our multidisciplinary clinic, patients with syn-dromic or bicoronal craniosynostosis (ie, Aperts or Crouzon syndrome) and associated minor suture craniosynostosis are offered either poste-rior cranial vault distraction or suturectomy and postoperative helmeting, depending on their age of presentation. Patients under the age of 6 months are treated with suturectomy and helmeting. Those above the age of 6 months are offered a posterior vault distraction (**Figs. 3** and **4**). These patients are then followed every 6 months for ophthalmologic evaluation for any signs of elevated intra-cranial pressure. Both techniques have been proven to offer beneficial management of cranial expansion as well as the normalization of cranial morphology (**Fig. 5**).

SAGITTAL/METOPIC CRANIOSYNOSTOSIS WITH ASSOCIATED SQUAMOUS SYNOSTOSIS (SCAPHOCEPHALY)

Patients with scaphocephaly and trigonocephaly are also managed within a multidisciplinary clinic. If

Cranial Volume Analysis

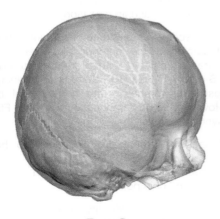
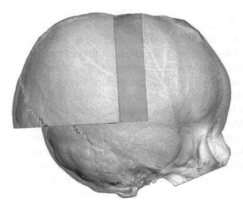

Pre-Op
940 cm³

Post-Op
1,092 cm³

Fig. 4. Preop and postop volume analysis.

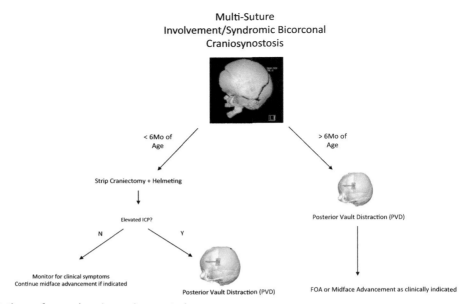

Multi-Suture Involvement/Syndromic Bicorconal Craniosynostosis

< 6Mo of Age

> 6Mo of Age

Strip Craniectomy + Helmeting

Elevated ICP?

N   Y

Monitor for clinical symptoms
Continue midface advancement if indicated

Posterior Vault Distraction (PVD)

Posterior Vault Distraction (PVD)

FOA or Midface Advancement as clinically indicated

Fig. 5. Pathway for syndromic craniosynostosis.

operative management is indicated before 6 months of age, patients are offered endoscopic suturectomy with postoperative helmeting. If patients present over 6 months of age they are offered a cranial expansion procedure (**Fig. 6**). There are numerous techniques used for the surgical treatment of scaphocephaly. In our practice we aim to address deformity by correcting the following:

1. Normalizing the occipital bullet (**Fig. 7**)
2. Correction of bitemporal narrowing
3. Decrease the AP dimension while increasing the biparietal width

We prefer to address the posterior 2/3rd of the scaphocephaly with a posterior cranial vault remodeling technique. From the prone approach, a posterior bandeau is created from the middle third of the cranium and expanded using a tongue and grove technique. This allows lifting of the occipital region as well as increasing the biparietal width (see **Fig. 7**). The posterior third of the calvarium is then fitted to create the vertex. In a study by Hopper and colleagues, they were able to quantify the frontal bossing correction with a single-stage middle and posterior vault expansion. Patients under the age of 1 showed consistent improvement of their frontal bossing within 2 years with an expansion procedure that was limited anteriorly to the coronal sutures[14]. If patients present with continued bitemporal narrowing or frontal bossing, a traditional fronto-orbital advancement with an interposition graft is usually indicated.

ANTERIOR PLAGIOCEPHALY ASSOCIATED WITH FRONTO-SPHENOID SYNOSTOSIS

Anterior plagiocephaly can be associated with deformational plagiocephaly as well as unicoronal craniosynostosis. In unicoronal craniosynostosis there is a consistent morphologic pattern consisting of:

1. flattening of the ipsilateral frontal and parietal bones and bossing of the contralateral forehead.
2. verticalization of the greater wind of the sphenoid leading to a superior orbital rim (harlequin deformity).
3. ipsilateral nasal root deviation
4. contralateral chin deviation

In recent years, numerous studies have well documented the anterior plagiocephaly differences associated with premature fusion of the FS suture.[15] Like UCS there is a flattening of the ipsilateral forehead with contralateral bossing. However, key differences were seen in FS suture synostosis involve:

1. lack of orbital rim elevation (no harlequin deformity)
2. contralateral nasal root deviation
3. midline chin point

It is important to identify these differences as the surgical technique should correct for the specific deformities. Surgical management should involve the utilization of a frontal-orbital advancement.

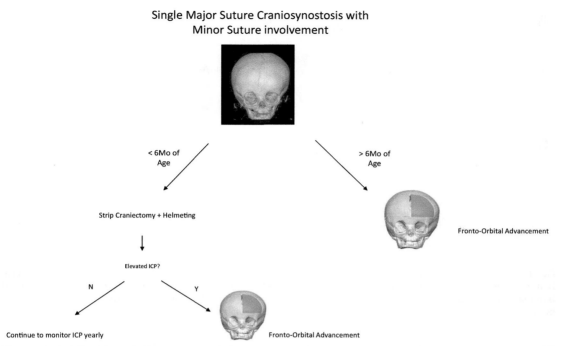

Fig. 6. Pathway for single suture craniosynostosis.

Mundinger and colleagues described their 12-year experience in managing patients with FS synostosis. Their 3D analysis of the ipsilateral FS orbit was characterized as more of a shallow trapezoid which was wide and short. In contrast, a UCS ipsilateral orbit was characterized as a tall, narrow, deep parallelogram (aka Harlequin deformity) (Fig. 8). In contrast to previously reported cases, the authors emphasize that the different orbital morphologies should alter the shaping of the frontal orbital bandeau. In the FS bandeau, balancing of the orbital brow should involve elevation and narrowing, as opposed to lowered and widened in the UCS bandeau (15) (Fig. 9). In many instances, we chose to perform an incomplete fronto-orbital bandeau. This involves performing an osteotomy within the orbital brow of the contralateral orbit. Advancement and hinging of the

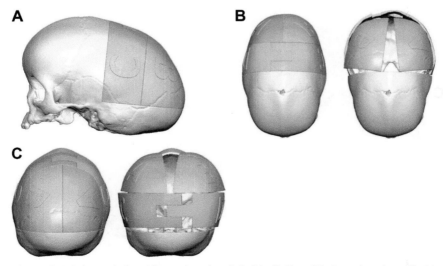

Fig. 7. (A): Patient wit scaphocephaly and associated occipital bulleting. (B). Superior view of a posterior vault reconstruction with creation of a posterior bandeau using the middle third of the cranium (C). Creation of the "tongue and groove" to allow for biparietal widening.

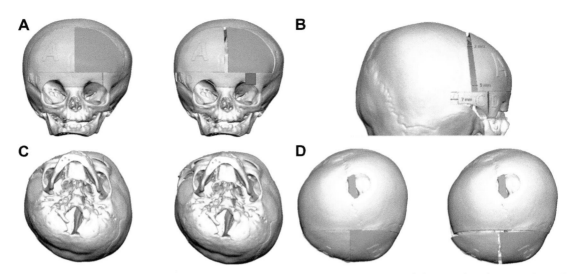

Fig. 8. Correction of anterior plagiocephaly with a frontal-orbital advancement. (*A*). Note that the contralateral bandeau ends in the orbital brow. Interpositional bone graft in blue. (*B–D*): Closing osteotomies of the ipsilateral bandeau at the lateral orbital rim allow for over correction of the orbital deformity and advancement of the brow.

bandeau on the ipsilateral side along the lateral orbital rim allow for the correction of the orbital deformity in height as width without disturbing the contralateral orbit. Over correction of the deformity on the ipsilateral side often requires an interpositional bone graft at the contralateral orbital brow (**Fig. 10**).

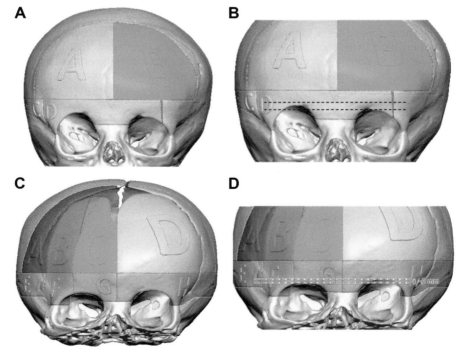

Fig. 9. Orbital Dysmorphology between Unicoronal Craniosynostosis (UCS) and Fronto-Sphenoid Craniosynostosis (FSC): (*A*). Right UCS (*B*). The dotted line represents the elevated superior orbital rim on the right (*C*). Right FCS (*D*). The inferior displaced superior orbital rim on the right.

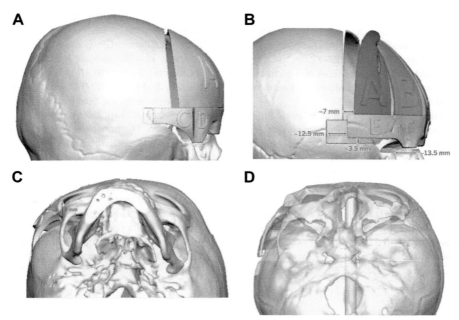

Fig. 10. Planned correction for UCS and FSC. (*A, C*). Overcorrection of UCS (*B, D*): Over Correction of FSC. Note the elevation of the temporal extension of the bandeau.

SUMMARY

Minor suture craniosynostosis is becoming recognized as a cause of intracranial pathology as well as alterations to cranial shape. Most of the cases do not occur in isolation, but in conjunction with another major suture synostosis. When it occurs in isolation, there is no dominant phenotype. Squamosal suture synostosis in isolation has been shown to present with scaphocephaly, plagiocephaly, or normocephaly. In patients who are normocephalic, and have no signs of elevated intracranial pressure, it is not advised to intervene. Patients who present with minor suture synostosis with involvement of a major suture, it should be managed by appropriate diagnosis, intracranial pressure evaluation, and surgical interventions to increase intracranial volume and normalize cranial shape. Postintervention management should include multidisciplinary care and yearly evaluations of intracranial pressure status.

CLINICS CARE POINTS

- Frontosphenoidal (FS) craniosynostosis should be suspected in cases of anterior plagiocephaly without the involvement of the coronal sutures. Orbital shape and morphology should be accounted for in these cases.

- Correction of FS craniosynostosis should involve a frontal bandeau that seeks to elevate the superior orbital rim.

- Suspicion of minor suture craniosynostosis should warrant imaging as well as genetic workup as many published reports are multi-suture in nature.

DISCLOSURE

The authors have no relevant financial or nonfinancial relationships to disclose.

REFERENCES

1. Mehta VA, Bettegowda C, Jallo GI, et al. The evolution of surgical management for craniosynostosis. Neurosurg Focus 2010;29:E5.
2. Runyan CM, Xu MDW, Alperovich M, et al. Minor Suture Fusion in Syndromic Craniosynostosis. Plast Reconstr Surg 2017;140(3):434e–45e.
3. Wilkie AO, Byren JC, Hurst JA, et al. Prevalence and complications of single-gene and chromosomal disorders in craniosynostosis. Pediatrics 2010;126: e391–400.
4. van der Meulen J. Metopic synostosis. Childs Nerv Syst 2012;28(9):1359–67.
5. JM S Jr, Singh DJ, Reid RR, et al. Squamosal suture synostosis: a cause of atypical skull asymmetry. Plast Reconstr Surg 2012;130:165–76.

6. Chawla R, Alden TD, Bizhanova A, et al. Squamosal suture craniosynostosis due to hyperthyroidism caused by an activating thyrotropin receptor mutation (T632I). Thyroid 2015;25:1167–72.

7. Doumit GD, Sidaoui J, Meisler E, et al. Squamosal suture craniosynostosis in Muenke syndrome. J Craniofac Surg 2014;25:429–31.

8. Cho DY, Evans KN, Weed MC, et al. Bilateral Squamosal Suture Craniosynostosis Presenting with Abducens Nerve Palsy and Severe Papilledema. World Neurosurg 2020;138:344–8.

9. Mazzaferro DM, Naran S, Wes AM, et al. Incidence of cranial base suture fusion in infants with craniosynostosis. Plast Reconstr Surg 2018;141:559 e–570e.

10. Ranger A, Chaudhary N, Matic D. Craniosynostosis involving the squamous temporal sutures. J Craniofac Surg 2010;21:1547–50.

11. Greene AK, Mulliken JB, Proctor MR, et al. Phenotypically unusual combined craniosynostoses: presentation and management. Plast Reconstr Surg 2008;122:853–62.

12. Eley KA, Thomas GP, Sheerin F, et al. The Significance of Squamosal Suture Synostosis. J Craniofac Surg 2016;27(6):1543–9.

13. Persing JA. MOC-PS(SM) CME article: management considerations in the treatment of craniosynostosis. Plast Reconstr Surg 2008;121:1–11.

14. Khechoyan D, Schook C, Birgfeld CB, et al. Changes in frontal morphology after single-stage open posterior-middle vault expansion for sagittal craniosynostosis. Plast Reconstr Surg. 2012 Feb; 129(2):504-516. doi: 10.1097/PRS. 0b013e31823aec1d.

15. Puente-Espel J, Kozusko SD, Konofaos P, et al. Isolated Frontosphenoidal Suture Craniosynostosis: Treatment Approaches and Literature Review for a Unique Condition. J Craniofac Surg. 2020 Jun;31(4): e385-e388. doi: 10.1097/SCS.0000000000006349.

Syndromic Craniosynostosis
Cranial Vault Expansion in Infancy

Sameer Shakir, MD, Craig B. Birgfeld, MD*

KEYWORDS

- Complex craniosynostosis • Craniofacial syndromes • Acrocephalosyndactyly • Apert • Crouzon
- Muenke • Pfeiffer • Saethre-Chotzen

KEY POINTS

- The fundamental goal of cranial vault reconstruction in syndromic craniosynostosis (CS) is to increase the intracranial volume to improve cerebral blood flow and prevent sequelae of increased intracranial pressure (iICP), while normalizing the dysmorphology of the skull, orbits, and midface with as few operations as possible.
- Early surgical intervention may facilitate corneal protection and alleviate iICP; however, later intervention may result in less bony relapse and need for additional surgery.
- CS frequently presents with cephalocranial disproportion and venous hypertension in the setting of posterior cranial fossa constriction, potentially leading to iICP, hydrocephalus, and/or Chiari type I malformations.
- Compared with anterior cranial expansion, posterior expansion increases intracranial volume to a greater degree while potentially delaying or obviating the need for fronto-orbital advancement or monobloc fronto-facial advancement until a later age when bone thickness and orbital morphology are more favorable.

OVERVIEW

Syndromic craniosynostosis (CS) represents a relatively uncommon disease process that poses significant reconstructive challenges for the craniofacial surgeon. Although there is considerable overlap in clinical features associated with various forms of syndromic CS, key extracranial features and close examination of the extremities help to distinguish the subtypes (**Table 1** and **Fig. 1**). While Virchow's law can easily guide the diagnosis of single suture, nonsyndromic CS, syndromic CS traditionally results in atypical presentations inherent to multiple suture fusion. Coronal ring involvement in isolation or associated with additional suture fusion is the most common pattern in syndromic CS often resulting in turribrachycephaly.[1]

GOALS OF TREATMENT AND FUNCTIONAL ISSUES

The fundamental goal of cranial vault remodeling (CVR) in CS is to increase the intracranial volume to improve cerebral blood flow and prevent increased intracranial pressure (iICP), while normalizing the dysmorphology of the skull, orbits, and midface. Limiting the total number of interventions to achieve this goal remains challenging as these children present with severe deformities, low physiologic reserve, and future growth potential.[2] While the timing of initial intervention remains debated, there are several considerations that inform this decision. Beyond identifying the craniofacial dysmorphology in patients with syndromic CS, the initial evaluation must first assess for life-threatening comorbidities related to airway

University of Washington, Seattle Children's Hospital, M/S OB.9.532, PO Box 5371, 4800 Sand Point Way, Seattle, WA 98105, USA
* Corresponding author.
E-mail address: craig.birgfeld@seattlechildrens.org

Oral Maxillofacial Surg Clin N Am 34 (2022) 443–458
https://doi.org/10.1016/j.coms.2022.01.006
1042-3699/22/© 2022 Elsevier Inc. All rights reserved.

Table 1
Syndromic craniosynostosis classification

Syndrome	Gene; Inheritance; Incidence	Phenotype (Headshape, Orbits, Midface)	Phenotype (Associated Anomalies)	Neurocognition
Apert	FGFR2 AD or de novo 1/65,000–1/88,000	• Turribrachycephaly (bicoronal CS) • Large AF with short ACF • High, flat forehead with transverse frontal skin furrow • Shallow orbits with ocular proptosis, horizontal grooves above supraorbital ridges, mild hypertelorism, and down-slanting palpebral fissures • Severe midface hypoplasia with anterior open bite and high arched or cleft palate • Psittichorhina (ie, "Parrot beak" nasal deformity)	• Bilateral symmetric syndactyly of the hands and feet • Syndactyly in form of "mitten," "spade," or "rosebud" hand • Deficient first webspce • Radial clinodactyly • Acne vulgaris during adolescence • Gut malrotation	• Developmental delay • Severe intellectual disability
Crouzon	FGFR2 AD or de novo 1.6/100,000	• Progressive multisuture CS • Acrobrachycephaly (bicoronal CS ± sagittal, lambdoid, metopic CS) • Shallow orbits with exorbitism, ocular proptosis, mild hypertelorism • Midface hypoplasia with high arched, constricted palate and anterior open bite • Psittichorhina (ie, "Parrot beak" nasal deformity)	• PDA, aortic coarctation • Low-set ears, ear canal malformations, hearing loss	• Normal
Muenke	FGFR3 AD or de novo 1/30,000	• Unicoronal CS (anterior plagiocephaly) vs bicoronal CS (brachycephaly) • Rare midface hypoplasia	• Thimble-like middle phalanges • Hearing loss	• Intellectual disability • Deafness

Saethre-Chotzen	TWIST1 AD or de novo 1/50,000	• Heterogeneous pattern of CS • Unicoronal CS (anterior plagiocephaly), bicoronal CS (brachycephaly), ± lambdoid CS (acrocephaly) • Ptosis, hypertelorism, strabismus, epicanthal folds • Facial asymmetry, low-set hairline • Cleft palate with high arch • Psittichorhina (ie, "Parrot beak" nasal deformity) with nasal septal deviation	• Congenital heart defects • Brachydactyly, syndactyly, clinodactyly • Broad thumb/hallux with valgus deformity	• Usually normal with reports of mild to moderate intellectual disability
Pfeiffer	Type I: FGFR2; AD Type II: FGFR1; de novo Type III: FGFR1, de novo	Type I (Bicoronal [Turribrachycephaly]) • Exorbitism, hypertelorism, strabismus, down-slanting palpebral fissures • Moderate midface hypoplasia with anterior open bite and cleft palate • Psittichorhina (ie, "Parrot beak" nasal deformity) Type II (Kleeblattschädel [bicoronal, sagittal, lambdoid]) • Severe ocular proptosis • Moderate midface hypoplasia Type III (Pancraniosynostosis [turribrachycephaly]) • No kleeblattschädel • Short ACF • Shallow orbits with severe ocular proptosis • Moderate – severe midface hypoplasia	• ASD, PS, ToF • Broad thumbs/hallux • Simple syndactyly • Gut malrotation	• Type 1 normal • Type 2 & 3 variable

Data from Taylor JA, Bartlett SP. What's New in Syndromic Craniosynostosis Surgery? Plast Reconstr Surg. 2017;140(1):82e-93e and Sawh-Martinez R, Steinbacher DM. Syndromic Craniosynostosis. Clin Plast Surg. 2019;46(2):141-155.

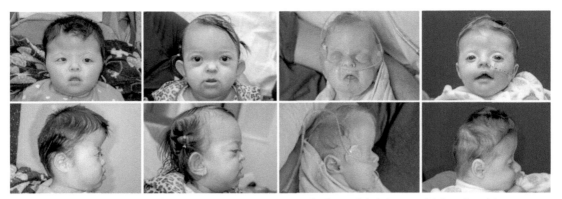

Fig. 1. Varying presentations of syndromic craniosynostosis. (Left to right) 2-year-old female with Apert syndrome resulting in turribrachycephaly, exorbitism, mild hypertelorism, and midface retrusion. 12-month-old female presenting with Crouzon syndrome resulting in brachycephaly, exorbitism, and midface hypoplasia. 4-week-old female with Pfeiffer syndrome characterized by Kleeblattschädel deformity, severe ocular proptosis, and moderate–severe midface hypoplasia. 3-month-old female with Saethre-Chotzen syndrome characterized by turribrachycephaly and prominent frontal bulge, mild blepharoptosis, and psittichorhina.

obstruction, cardiopulmonary function, and feeding issues. These diagnoses even supersede underlying iICP, as it is thought that the existing open sutures compensate for brain growth in the interim.[3]

Airway

There is a low threshold for polysomnography to diagnose central or obstructive sleep apnea (OSA) in children with syndromic CS who present with midface hypoplasia-related noisy breathing and/or snoring. OSA may be initially managed with the use of continuous positive airway pressure (CPAP) masks and adenotonsillectomies, while less common central sleep apnea may be secondary to underlying Chiari I deformation causing brain stem compression. As the midface hypoplasia observed in syndromic CS typically worsens with age, so does the incidence of airway compromise.[4] Temporary tracheostomies should be considered in patients who fail conservative measures. Although some centers will consider early frontofacial advancement to address the midface hypoplasia and avoid tracheostomy, we believe that the data remain unconvincing in the setting of technical complexity, high complication rates, and inconsistent results. Contrastingly, tracheostomy offers reliable airway protection with high efficacy, technical ease, and a limited complication profile.[5]

INTRACRANIAL PRESSURE

Causes of iICP include cephalocranial disproportion (CCD), hydrocephalus, venous hypertension, anomalous venous drainage, and OSA. CCD represents a mismatch between intracranial contents and volumetric space. Chronically iICP leads to impaired myelination and is associated with poor neurodevelopment as devastating consequences include optic nerve atrophy leading to blindness and psychomotor delay. Reports by Renier and colleagues quoted the incidence of iICP at 45%, 62.5%, and 29% in Apert, Crouzon, and other forms of syndromic CS, respectively.[6] Although it remains unknown for how long or how high ICP must be elevated before causing permanent detrimental effects on neurocognitive function, the rate of iICP in syndromic CS most accurately approaches 50% when directly measured by invasive overnight intracranial monitoring.[1]

The clinical presentation of iICP in young children includes compensatory brain and skull growth in nonfused regions resulting in characteristic skull changes. Clinical signs and symptoms include multiple unexpected cranial defects, suture diastasis, bulging fontanels, increasing head circumference, raised collar of bone around the fontanel (ie, "volcano sign"), endocranial "thumb-printing," small/large ventricles, erosions of the sella turcica, and papilledema.[1,3] Additional findings include ventriculomegaly (~40%), venous drainage anomalies, and OSA. The real-world diagnosis of iICP relies on secondary assessments including physical exam to assess dural tension, serial head circumference measurements to assess changes in growth curves, MRI to monitor for central nervous system abnormalities, and noninvasive papilledema testing. However, iICP can be difficult to assess in this patient population as the sensitivity of papilledema as a prognosticator for iICP remains low in children less than 8 years of age.[7]

Hydrocephalus, Ventriculoperitoneal Shunting, and Chiari Malformations

While the treatment of CS aims to increase ICV, the treatment of hydrocephalus aims to decrease ICV by reducing the size of the cerebral ventricles. The sequence of treatment depends on the severity of hydrocephalus, as simultaneous treatment may limit ICV expansion due to CSF shunting.[6] In general, severe or progressive hydrocephalus requires initial shunting. Cranial expansion may proceed once the ventricles remain stable in size. If there is mild or slowly progressive hydrocephalus, cranial expansion may be performed and the need for subsequent shunting reassessed using postoperative imaging.

Chari malformations are reported in approximately 30%, 70%, and 100% of newborns with Apert, Crouzon, and Pfeiffer syndrome, respectively.[5,8,9] The diagnosis carries the risk of noncommunicating hydrocephalus resulting in syringomyelia, impaired coordination, paralysis, disordered swallowing, and central sleep apnea, which may be fatal. MRI remains a critical imaging modality in patients with syndromic CS and Chiari malformations. Repeat imaging is often indicated following cranial expansion, as these patients may subsequently demonstrate noncommunicating hydrocephalus. Whether or not Chiari malformations in syndromic CS represent an acquired phenomenon continues to be debated. Proponents cite an increased rate of Chiari malformations in patients with small posterior fossa related to lambdoid suture fusion and disproportional hindbrain growth, while opponents cite equivocal rates of malformations independent of posterior fossa volume.[10] While the definitive management of a Chiari malformation is direct neurosurgical decompression, some centers offer prophylactic treatment of asymptomatic malformations through posterior cranial expansion with or without foramen magnum decompression (**Fig. 2**).[11–13]

Ocular

Approximately 50% of children with syndromic CS suffer from some degree of visual impairment, with amblyopia and ametropia representing the most common diagnoses.[1] Underlying bone and soft-tissue anomalies result in exorbitism and ocular proptosis that cause lagophthalmos, progress to corneal desiccation, and potentially blindness. Underlying iICP may lead to optic nerve atrophy. While frontofacial advancement eventually treats

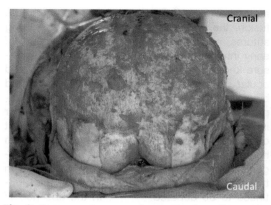

Fig. 2. Foramen magnum decompression. Open posterior cranial vault expansion with the removal of bone flap, occipital barrel stave osteotomies, and decompression of the foramen magnum. Note cerebellar and brainstem decompression following removal of the occipital bone down to the foramen magnum. The white arrow represents the torcula.

the underlying pathology, temporary tarsorrhaphies provide interval ocular protection.

Neurodevelopmental

Proponents of early repair (ie, under 1 year of age) argue patients may demonstrate higher developmental scores including intelligence quotient (IQ), while opponents of early interventions fail to find a similar correlation and believe head shape correction to be better maintained in the long-term when delaying surgery (ie, over 1 year of age).[14–18] Patients with CS are at risk for neurodevelopmental delay—whether this can be modified through surgery and the optimal timing of surgery continues to be debated. Perhaps the complex relationship can be succinctly summarized by the following: (1) there is a correlation between the number of sutures fused and iICP, (2) iICP inversely correlates with neurocognitive function, and (3) operative intervention reduces ICP.

INTERVENTIONS
Surgical Timing

CVR in syndromic CS can reliably lower iICP; however, there is a high recurrence rate.[19] There is significant variability in the timing of surgical approaches due to a lack of rigorous outcomes data. A 2006 poll conducted during the meeting of the International Society of Craniofacial Surgery (ISCFS) noted that most of the members perform some sort of operative intervention within the first year of life.[20] The key considerations in timing operative repair include long-term morphometric outcomes and neurodevelopment. Secondary factors include single versus multiple suture fusion, the presence of adjacent decompressing sutures, and phenotypic severity. Proponents of early intervention cite the need to prevent exposure keratopathy in the setting of exorbitism and ocular proptosis and to expand the constricted brain in the setting of iICP.[17] Worsening turricephaly may serve as a relative indication for earlier intervention as excessively increased skull height can be difficult to correct later. Beyond long-term head-shape correction, existing literature suggests improved neurodevelopment outcomes in the early intervention cohort, although this continues to be debated.[6,14,21,22] In the absence of iICP, however, delaying surgery beyond 1 year of age likely produces a more stable morphometric result with decreased need for subsequent revision.[8,10] Not only must early intervention contend with thinner, less rigid cranial bone, but also with a rapidly enlarging brain that may quickly fill the expanded intracranial space and recapitulate brachycephaly. Through various long-term analyses of head-shape correction in single-suture CS, multiple high-volume centers have demonstrated that cranial growth does not normalize postoperatively.[23,24] Utria and colleagues reported patients undergoing intervention before 6 months of age were 4.1 times likelier to undergo a subsequent major reoperation based on Whitaker classification.[25]

Anterior Versus Posterior

Anterior-first interventions aimed to achieve early corneal protection in the setting of exorbitism and frontal retrusion. However, long-term data suggest these anterior advancements tended to require reoperations for both functional and morphometric concerns—especially when performed before age 6 months.[26–28] In a series of syndromic patients undergoing fronto-orbital advancement (FOA), Wall and colleagues reported a reoperative rate of 8.2%, which doubled to 16.7% in patients with Apert syndrome.[28] Posterior-first techniques including various open and less invasive occipital cranioplasties offer a greater expansion of the ICV, may delay/obviate the need for additional anterior expansion to a later age that is associated with increased bony stability and may preclude the need for foramen magnum decompression in patients with Chiari type I malformations.[13,29,30] Nevertheless, in patients with Chiari malformations and a pre-existing VPS, posterior cranial expansion with suboccipital decompression of the foramen magnum is typically performed to avoid life-threatening complications stemming from shunt failure.[3]

Major drawbacks of posterior techniques include anomalous transosseous venous drainage that may lead to mortality if indiscriminately ligated, technically challenging dural dissection that risks significant bleeding from the torcula, and newborn supine positioning that not only limits the amount of achievable postoperative expansion but also remains entirely reliant on the strength of the implanted hardware.[2,31] While there are several advantages to a posterior-first approach, patients presenting with severe exorbitism and frontofacial retrusion will require temporary tarsorrhaphies to prevent corneal ulceration until an anterior expansion is performed.[1] Nevertheless, both anterior and posterior techniques continue to be used for differing indications in syndrome-specific protocols that attempt to minimize the total number of surgical interventions, iICP, and relapse.

Strip Craniectomy

Strip craniectomy in isolation does not replace the need for subsequent cranial expansion; however, it may be necessary to reduce life-threatening sequela of severe CCD during the neonatal period (**Fig. 3**). Existing data suggest early craniectomy may delay the need for subsequent cranial expansion to a more appropriate age.[32] Neonates with the W290 C pathogenic variant typically seen in FGFR2-related mutations and anomalous venous drainage represent severely affected subsets benefiting from early craniectomy and presenting with hydrocephalus requiring shunting.[33] When left untreated, there may erosive changes, thinning, and progressive loss of cranial bone from underlying brain growth and compensatory overexpansion in low resistance regions of the calvaria including the fontanels and patent minor sutures. Thickened bony constriction bands develop in the regions of highest resistance extending from the pterion to the vertex. Utilizing a conventional bicoronal incision, these bony constrictions are identified and released, temporarily relieving iICP. Subsequent bony regeneration occurs through signaling from the osteogenic dura in a similar fashion to free-floating cranial vault release procedures.[31,33]

Serving as an alternative to open CVR procedures, endoscopic strip craniectomy with postoperative helmet therapy (ESC + PHT) may be performed during the first year of life.[34,35] When performed between 1 and 4 months of age in patients with bicoronal CS, the Boston group reported significant improvements in head shape and slowing of progressive turricephaly, although over 50% of the cohort ultimately required anterior

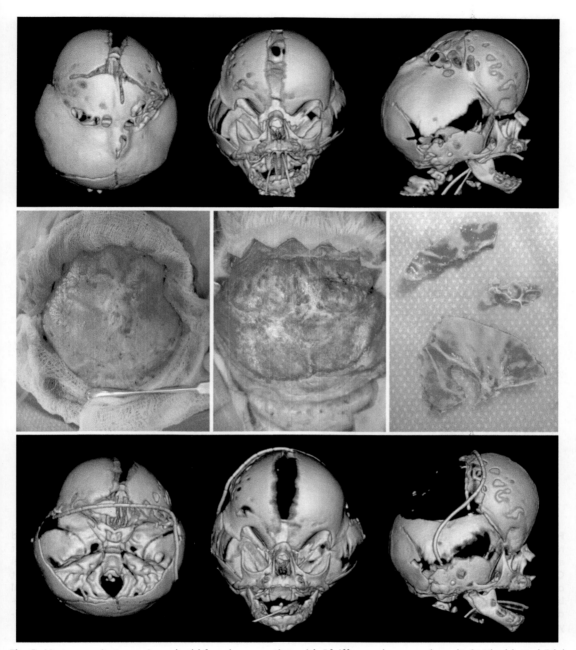

Fig. 3. Vertex craniectomy. 4-week-old female presenting with Pfeiffer syndrome and resultant Kleeblattschädel deformity found to have severe constriction in the center portion of the skull with multiple areas of transosseous brain herniation and thin bone. She underwent a wide vertex craniectomy and barrel stave osteotomies.

expansion in the form of FOA within a short follow-up period. Nevertheless, their low rate of reported morbidity warrants consideration.[34,35]

Fronto-Orbital Advancement

In less severe cases of CCD primarily associated with severe frontal retrusion and exorbitism, FOA

or early monobloc may increase ICV and protect the globes. When performed prior to 6 months of age, however, McCarthy et al. reported relapse rates greater than 33% in syndromic patients undergoing FOA.[36] Our institutional practice has been to perform FOA closer to 2 years of age to take advantage of stiffer bone that allows for a more stable long-term advancement (**Fig. 4**). The

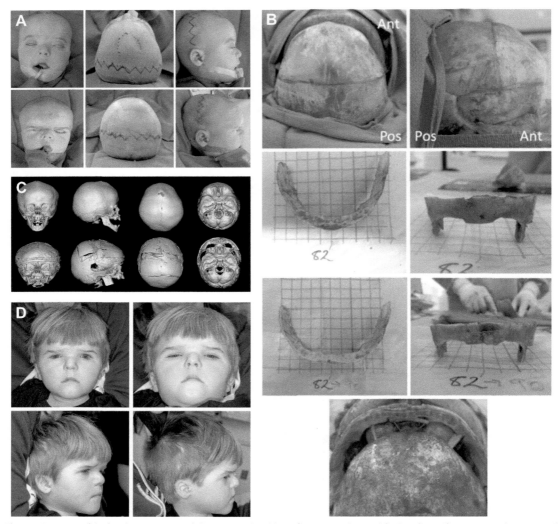

Fig. 4. Fronto-orbital advancement. (*A*) 11-month-old male presenting with Saethre–Chotzen syndrome and resultant turribrachycephaly and volcano sign (dotted circle). He underwent FOA and bilateral canthopexies at age 15 months. (*B*) Subperiosteal dissection of the cranial vault, creation of the orbital bandeau with lateral C-shaped osteotomies, widening of the mid-bandeau using interposition bone grafts at the nasion, placement of bone grafts along the posterior aspect of the bandeau for additional stability, and placement of cranial bone buttress grafts from the sphenoid to the bandeau along the orbital roof. (*C*) Preoperative (top) and immediate postoperative (bottom) imaging demonstrating presenting deformity and resultant expansion. (*D*) One-year postoperative presentation is consistent with a stable head shape correction.

techniques for FOA remain consistent across nonsyndromic and syndromic CS with 2 important caveats: (1) need for increased expansion, (2) varying bone quality. Many techniques exist for enlarging and subsequently stabilizing the frontal fossa including the tenon-type tongue-in-groove bandeau advocated by Fearon and colleagues[37] In general, the frontal bandeau must be advanced forward and inferiorly to in a stair-step manner to counteract postoperative supraorbital recession and elevation. Our institutional practice also

includes supraorbital bandeau expansion using an interposition bone graft, bilateral temporal tenons, C-shaped lateral orbital osteotomies, and simultaneous middle vault expansion to better address turricephaly (see **Fig. 1**). Fixation is performed using resorbable suture and plates, with autologous morselized bone graft used to fill cranial defects.[38] Our data suggest anterior vault surgery in this cohort represents a remodeling rather than a true expansion, with a decrease in anterior cranial height and circumferential expansion of the bandeau.[38] We recommend overcorrection of the supraorbital bandeau and forehead in the setting of relapse and decreased cranial growth. A criticism of concurrent middle vault expansion with craniotomy extending to the lambdoid sutures includes the inability to preserve unoperated biparietal bone for eventual autologous frontal cranioplasty at maturity.[3,10]

Early Monobloc

Monobloc advancement offers simultaneous cranial and subcranial decompression, circumferential orbital expansion with the correction of exorbitism, and midface advancement with improvement in OSA and malocclusion. Monobloc advancement is ideally performed around the 8 to 10 year age range to mitigate secondary bony relapse and injury to developing permanent maxillary molars.[39,40] Nevertheless, monobloc-first interventions may be considered in infants with iICP, severe exorbitism, and OSA (**Fig. 5**).[39] With the advent of distraction osteogenesis (DO), monobloc DO offers decreased morbidity and skeletal relapse owing to latency and activation periods that allow for adequate healing and dead space minimization in the prefrontal space through gradual advancement.[41]

Even in the most experienced hands, however, the procedure carries significant morbidity including persistent CSF leak, ascending infection, frontal bone necrosis, and death.[42] Arnaud and colleagues advocated for a pericranial flap to line the prefrontal space following transcranial osteotomy in an attempt to minimize serious complications.[42] Monobloc advancement becomes increasingly more complicated in infants under the age of 2 years who lose a greater portion of total blood volume and require secondary surgery stemming from postoperative midface growth arrest.[39,43,44] As the anterior skull base undergoes a progressive ossification after birth with the majority ossified by 3 years of age, the transcranial osteotomy must be carefully visualized along the anterior skull base.[45] Nassar and colleagues suggest a nasofrontal osteotomy for better visualization.[45] Lastly, early monobloc results in significant scar burden in the region of the pterygomaxillary junction that may increase the complexity of future subcranial movements including orthognathic surgery at skeletal maturity.[46,47]

Posterior Cranial Expansion

Given the inherent drawbacks of anterior approaches and for syndromic patients without indications for early monobloc, posterior CVR aims to correct posterior flattening while providing a space for brain expansion. With the realization that the mesodermal bones of the posterior cranial fossa offer increased growth potential compared with the anterior cranial fossa bones derived from neural crest, various studies not only began to demonstrate greater ICV expansion using posterior expansion techniques but also reduced rates of tonsillar herniation and papilledema.[13,30,48] Posterior-first interventions may halt progressive turricephaly, improve frontal dysmorphology, and delay or altogether avoid the need for future frontal expansion thereby limiting iatrogenic injury to anterior growth and ossification centers.[49] Disadvantages of posterior techniques include increased risk of bleeding associated with bone flap elevation overlying the torcula and postoperative deformational plagiocephaly in supine infants. In general, open PVR techniques involve the removal and reshaping of occipital and suboccipital bone. Although various geometric osteotomy patterns exist, they typically offer a single-stage correction that simultaneously addresses occipital flatness and expands the posterior cranial fossa.

Suboccipital Decompression

Posterior cranial fossa constriction with subsequent ICV reduction stemming from lambdoid and skull base suture fusion serves as a hallmark of syndromic CS. Subsequent restriction of the sagittal sinus and torcula produces venous hypertension, leading to anomalous posterior venous drainage, tonsillar herniation (ie, Chiari type I malformation), and noncommunicating hydrocephalus.[9] Fearon and colleagues previously described simultaneous PVR and suboccipital decompression (SOD) of the foramen magnum.[11] Abnormal venous drainage near the confluence of sinuses is left islanded to the surrounding bone. The subperiosteal dissection continues up to the lateral margins of the foramen magnum and a suboccipital craniectomy (sparing the bony islands) is performed without further elevation of the bone flap off the underlying dura mater. Additionally, a standard PVR cephalad to the suboccipital decompression is performed to increase the ICV. In their initial series of 19 patients undergoing PVR with SOD, Chiari malformations resolved in 35%, improved in 35%, and remained stable in 30%.[11]

Spring-Mediated Cranioplasty

Lauritzen's clinical description of implantable craniofacial springs introduced a dynamic, gradual head shape correction across various symmetric intracranial and subcranial pathologies.[50,51] The procedure requires minimal access without dural

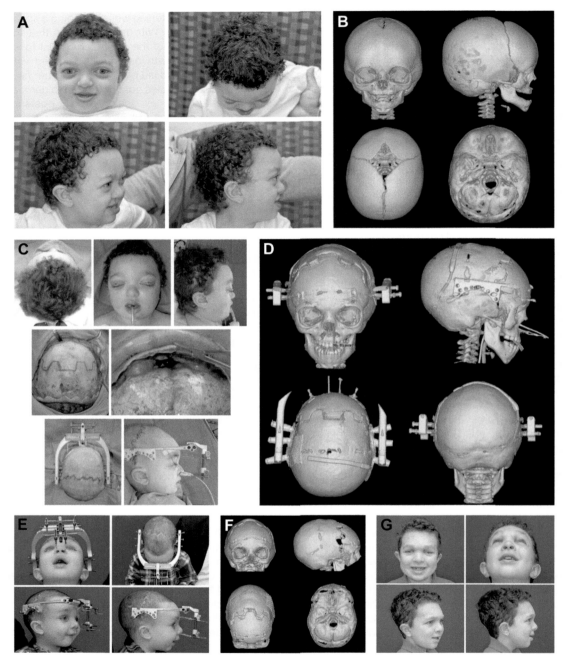

Fig. 5. Early monobloc advancement. (*A*, *B*) 3-year-old male with history of Crouzon syndrome and prior PVDO at 1 year of age presenting with frontal retrusion, exorbitism with exophthalmos, and midface hypoplasia in the setting of OSA. (*C*) Perioperative depiction of monobloc distraction involving temporary tarsorrhaphies in the setting of exorbitism, a tongue-and-groove bifrontal osteotomy pattern to maximize bone-to-bone contact during distraction, transcranial monobloc separation, and placement of an external Halo distractor device. (*D*) Immediate postoperative CT imaging depicts the FOA and Le Fort III osteotomy pattern and placement of unicortical halo fixation screws and bone anchoring midface fixation screws at the level of the supraorbital ridge and piriform rims. (*E*) At the end of consolidation, he presents with a stable anterior expansion with mild scaphocephaly, a symmetric brow position, an overcorrected midface with slight enophthalmos, and class I occlusal relations. (*F*, *G*) At 8.5 years of age, he presents with a stable cranial expansion, well-projected midface without exophthalmos, mild OSA requiring CPAP, and no signs or symptoms of iICP.

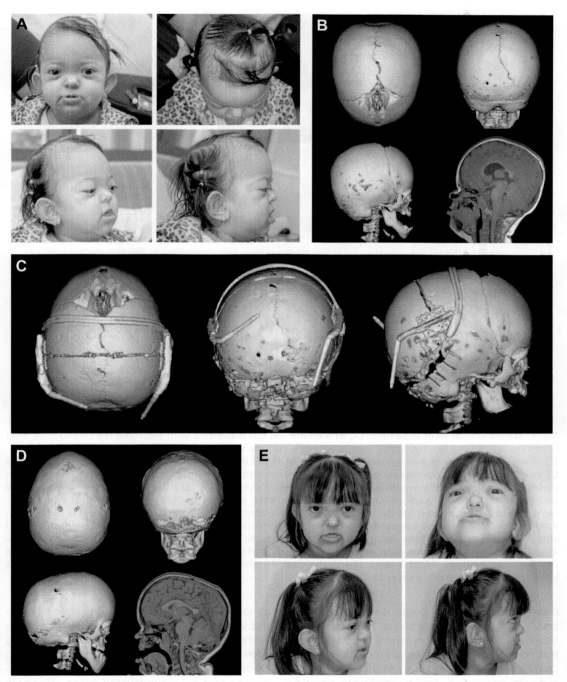

Fig. 6. Crouzon syndrome and Chiari malformation type 1. (*A*) 12-month-old female presenting with multisuture craniosynostosis, midface hypoplasia, and papilledema consistent with iICP in the setting of Crouzon syndrome. (*B*) Preoperative CT imaging notable for bilateral squamosal and left lambdoid suture fusion. MRI T1-weighted imaging notable for cerebellar tonsillar crowding, extension below the foramen magnum, effacement of CSF spaces, and a pointed shape most consistent with a Chiari type 1 malformation (*white arrow*). (*C*) Immediate post-operative CT imaging depicting PVDO with the placement of 2 semi-buried distractors, resorbable plate fixation across on open right lambdoid suture, and barrel-stave osteotomies along the basicranium. The patient underwent concurrent posterior fossa decompression with removal of bone down to the foramen magnum (center). (*D*) One-year postoperative CT imaging depicting stable expansion and resolution of the Chiari malformation (bottom right, *white arrow*). (*E*) At 2-years postoperative follow-up, she remains without iICP concerns.

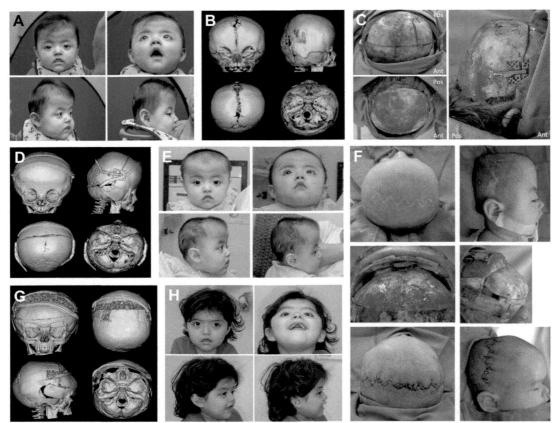

Fig. 7. Staged cranial vault expansion. (*A, B*) 8-month-old girl presenting with bicoronal craniosynostosis, mild hypertelorism, severe brachycephaly, and progressive turricephaly found to have Saethre–Chotzen syndrome. (*C*) Given her progressive turricephaly, she underwent PVDO at age 11 months. (*D*) Immediate postoperative CT imaging depicts the craniotomy pattern with the placement of 2 co-linear semi-buried distractors in the bi-parietal bones and barrel-stave osteotomies of the basal occipital bone. (*E*) After consolidation, she presented with improved turribrachycephaly and stable expansion of her posterior vault. (*F*) At age 22 months, she underwent FOA to further address her frontal dysmorphology related to remaining turribrachycephaly and Harlequin deformities. Closing-wedge osteotomies of bilateral superolateral orbits and onlay cranial bone grafts placed along the superior orbits of the bandeau helped to address the Harlequin deformities. (*G*) Immediate postoperative CT imaging demonstrates anterior expansion, lowering of the frontal bone to address turricephaly, and the new bandeau position. (*H*) At 3 years of age, she demonstrates a stable cranial expansion without significant brachycephalic relapse or concerns for iICP.

dissection, minimizing operative time and blood loss.[52] Compared with traditional PVR, there is a continued postoperative expansile force that may limit relapse due to an immediate increase in intracranial dead space resulting from single-stage, static reconstruction. Unlike semiburied devices used in PVDO, SMC offers an entirely subcutaneous hardware profile thereby limiting infection risk. The springs are anchored into the cranial bone across an osteotomy or open suture and apply a gradual expansile force until the force exerted by the spring reaches an equilibrium with the counteracting tissue forces.[12,50,51] The main drawbacks include a secondary procedure for hardware removal, inability to reshape contour abnormalities, and the inability to accurately predict the degree of postoperative expansion. While spring outcomes for nonsyndromic indications such as the correction of scaphocephaly seem to be dependent on a younger age at surgery, multiple groups have demonstrated spring efficacy in the syndromic patient population for children older than 12 months.[12,51]

The Great Ormond Street Hospital (GOSH) experience using SMC for posterior vault expansion similarly highlights a safe, effective head shape correction.[12] They utilize a sinusoidal bicoronal osteotomy beginning 5 cm posterior to the skin incision and terminating above or below the torcula depending on underlying venous anatomy. The degree of dural dissection near the torcula and foramen magnum is dependent on the degree of posterior bone flap mobility achieved. If inadequate bone flap mobility is noted, the bone flap may be elevated free of the dural attachments and reattached using steel wires before spring placement. Two springs are typically placed 2 cm from midline along the craniotomy edge and a posterior-based pericranial flap is draped over the springs before scalp closure. Over a 12-year experience, the authors reported a 97%

improvement in iICP in a cohort of 120 patients with syndromic CS at median age of 21 months.

Posterior Vault Distraction Osteogenesis

The introduction of PVDO revolutionized treatment algorithms of patients with syndromic CS.[53] Compared with other posterior techniques potentially limited by the soft tissue envelope and relapse related to supine positioning and an acute increase in postoperative intracranial dead space,

Table 2
Treatment protocol for syndromic craniosynostosis at Seattle Children's Hospital

Age	Intervention
Prenatal • Genetic counseling • Ultrasound evaluation • Delivery plan (Cesarean section)	
Postnatal • Airway obstruction, multilevel • OSA • Exposure keratopathy • Feeding issues • CCD with iICP • Cervical spine malformation • Genetic testing and counseling	• Tracheostomy • Polysomnography, CPAP, T&A • Temporary tarsorrhaphy • Gastrotomy tube • Strip craniectomy
3–6 mo • Hydrocephalus, Chiari malformation	• VPS
4–9 mo • Cranial morphology assessment	• PVDO
1–3 y • Cranial morphology assessment for frontal retrusion, exorbitism, midface retrusion, OSA	• FOA vs monobloc DO (early)
3–4 y • Large cranial defects	• Autologous bone grafting vs CAD/CAM alloplastic cranioplasty
6–12 y • Facial imbalance, exorbitism • Midface hypoplasia, exorbitism • Hypertelorism • Frontotemporal deformity	• Monobloc DO (ideal) • Le Fort III vs Le Fort II advancement with zygomatic repositioning • Box osteotomies, facial bipartition, subcranial medial orbital translocation • Onlay bone graft vs CAD/CAM alloplastic cranioplasty
Skeletal maturity • Skeletal malocclusion/(bi)maxillary retrognathism • Malar deficiency • Nasal deformity • Periorbital deformity	• Le Fort I osteotomy, bilateral sagittal split osteotomies, osseous genioplasty • Malar alloplastic augmentation, fat grafting • Open rhinoplasty • Canthoplasty/canthopexy

An ideal, staged cranial expansion approach used at our institution.
Abbreviations: CCD, cephalocranial disproportion; iICP, increased intracranial pressure; OSA, obstructive sleep apnea; DO, distraction osteogenesis, PVDO, posterior vault distraction osteogenesis; CPAP, continuous positive airway pressure; T&A, tonsilloadenoidectomy; VPS, ventriculoperitoneal shunt; FOA, fronto-orbital advancement; CAD/CAM, computer-aided design/computer-aided manufacturing.
Adapted from Forrest CR, Hopper RA. Craniofacial syndromes and surgery. Plast Reconstr Surg. 2013;131(1):86e-109e.

PVDO offers a tension-free, gradual bony expansion associated with overlying soft tissue stretch while maintaining vascularity to the bony transport segment.[54] Proponents cite low complication rates comparable to other posterior expansion techniques, comparative increase in ICV, favorable frontal morphology changes, potential resolution of Chiari type I malformations, and ability to delay and/or obviate additional frontal surgery (**Figs. 6** and **7**).[48,49,55] Certain centers use PVDO as the primary intervention in all patients with syndromic CS.[2,56] Drawbacks of PVDO include a largely uni-vector expansion instead of a three-dimensional change, hardware failure related to device loosening or separation from the bone-distraction interface, increased infection profile associated with semiburied devices, increased cutaneous scarring, inability to adjust distraction vectors postoperatively, and dural injuries further perpetuated during activation resulting from screw fixation/migration.[57]

The procedure involves a circumferential osteotomy extending from the mid-parietal region anteriorly, below the torcula inferiorly, and below the squamosal sutures laterally. A "tongue-in-groove" osteotomy pattern may be used to maximize bony stability. The bone flap remains adherent to the underlying dura, which minimizes intraoperative blood loss and maintains vascularity. Low occipital barrel stave osteotomies with greenstick outfractures may be lagged to the transport segment to further minimize bony step-off following distraction. Two semi-buried, self-ratcheting distractors are placements in a parasagittal, colinear position with a posterior or posterior–inferior vector depending on the degree of turricephaly. A transverse component may be considered in normocephalic patients with complex CS to achieve a multi-vector expansion. To prevent asymmetric expansion and bony instability, patent lambdoid sutures may be fixated using resorbable plating systems or sutures although this poses its own risks related to subsequent cranial growth (see **Fig. 6**). Distractor arms are typically placed anteriorly to prevent hardware failure with supine positioning. While several distraction protocols exist, traditional latency phases range from 5 to 7 days and activation proceeds at 0.5 to 2.0 mm (mm) daily followed by 2 to 3 months of consolidation.

SEATTLE CHILDREN'S PROTOCOL

Cranial expansion protocols in syndromic CS may follow an expectant or staged approach with the understanding that the first intervention is typically performed before age 1 year.[20] An expectant approach uses clinical and/or objective measures of iICP to guide the timing of intervention.[58] A staged approach analyzes a given patient's phenotype and offers interventions at predetermined time points.[1,30,49] Although staged approaches are more predictable, they may result in increased total number of procedures performed when considering the actual incidence of iICP at each stage. While there are some caveats related to longitudinal care that are beyond the scope of this article, **Table 2** presents an ideal, staged cranial expansion approach used at our institution.

CLINICS CARE POINTS

- In syndromic cases with Chiari type I malformations and constricted posterior cranial fossae, we perform PVDO with concurrent foramen magnum decompression.
- One challenge in syndromic CS management relates to the inability to clearly identify presenting phenotypes that would benefit from early monobloc advancement versus those who would benefit from staged FOA and subsequent Le Fort III advancement.
- To minimize relapse associated with early anterior expansion, we perform initial FOA at age ~2 years with subsequent subcranial surgery in adolescence.

REFERENCES

1. Forrest CR, Hopper RA. Craniofacial syndromes and surgery. Plast Reconstr Surg 2013;131(1):86e–109e.
2. Taylor JA, Bartlett SP. What's New in Syndromic Craniosynostosis Surgery? Plast Reconstr Surg 2017; 140(1):82e–93e.
3. Fearon JA. *Syndromic craniosynostosis, Neligan's Plastic surgery.* Vol 3. Fourth edition. London: Elsevier; 2018.
4. Patel N, Fearon JA. Treatment of the syndromic midface: a long-term assessment at skeletal maturity. Plast Reconstr Surg 2015;135(4):731e–42e.
5. Fearon JA, Rhodes J. Pfeiffer syndrome: a treatment evaluation. Plast Reconstr Surg 2009;123(5): 1560–9.
6. Renier D, Lajeunie E, Arnaud E, et al. Management of craniosynostoses. Childs Nerv Syst 2000;16(10–11):645–58.
7. Tuite GF, Chong WK, Evanson J, et al. The effectiveness of papilledema as an indicator of raised

intracranial pressure in children with craniosynostosis. Neurosurgery 1996;38(2):272–8.

8. Fearon JA, Podner C. Apert syndrome: evaluation of a treatment algorithm. Plast Reconstr Surg 2013; 131(1):132–42.

9. Cinalli G, Renier D, Sebag G, et al. Chronic tonsillar herniation in Crouzon's and Apert's syndromes: the role of premature synostosis of the lambdoid suture. J Neurosurg 1995;83(4):575–82.

10. Fearon JA. Evidence-based medicine: Craniosynostosis. Plast Reconstr Surg 2014;133(5):1261–75.

11. Scott WW, Fearon JA, Swift DM, et al. Suboccipital decompression during posterior cranial vault remodeling for selected cases of Chiari malformations associated with craniosynostosis. J Neurosurg Pediatr 2013;12(2):166–70.

12. Breakey RWF, van de Lande LS, Sidpra J, et al. Spring-assisted posterior vault expansion-a single-centre experience of 200 cases. Childs Nerv Syst 2021;37(10):3189–97.

13. Lin LO, Zhang RS, Hoppe IC, et al. Onset and Resolution of Chiari Malformations and Hydrocephalus in Syndromic Craniosynostosis following Posterior Vault Distraction. Plast Reconstr Surg 2019;144(4):932–40.

14. Arnaud E, Meneses P, Lajeunie E, et al. Postoperative mental and morphological outcome for nonsyndromic brachycephaly. Plast Reconstr Surg 2002; 110(1):6–12.

15. Starr JR, Kapp-Simon KA, Cloonan YK, et al. Presurgical and postsurgical assessment of the neurodevelopment of infants with single-suture craniosynostosis: comparison with controls. J Neurosurg 2007;107(2 Suppl):103–10.

16. Renier D, Arnaud E, Cinalli G, et al. Prognosis for mental function in Apert's syndrome. J Neurosurg 1996;85(1):66–72.

17. Hashim PW, Patel A, Yang JF, et al. The effects of whole-vault cranioplasty versus strip craniectomy on long-term neuropsychological outcomes in sagittal craniosynostosis. Plast Reconstr Surg 2014;134(3):491–501.

18. Da Costa AC, Walters I, Savarirayan R, et al. Intellectual outcomes in children and adolescents with syndromic and nonsyndromic craniosynostosis. Plast Reconstr Surg 2006;118(1):175–81.

19. Spruijt B, Joosten KFM, Driessen C, et al. Algorithm for the Management of Intracranial Hypertension in Children with Syndromic Craniosynostosis. Plast Reconstr Surg 2015;136(2):331–40.

20. Mathijssen IM. Guideline for Care of Patients With the Diagnoses of Craniosynostosis: Working Group on Craniosynostosis. J Craniofac Surg 2015;26(6): 1735–807.

21. Patel A, Yang JF, Hashim PW, et al. The impact of age at surgery on long-term neuropsychological outcomes in sagittal craniosynostosis. Plast Reconstr Surg 2014;134(4):608e–17e.

22. van der Vlugt JJB, van der Meulen J, van den Braak R, et al. Insight into the Pathophysiologic Mechanisms behind Cognitive Dysfunction in Trigonocephaly. Plast Reconstr Surg 2017;139(4):954e–64e.

23. Fearon JA, Ruotolo RA, Kolar JC. Single sutural craniosynostoses: surgical outcomes and long-term growth. Plast Reconstr Surg 2009;123(2):635–42.

24. Seruya M, Oh AK, Boyajian MJ, et al. Long-term outcomes of primary craniofacial reconstruction for craniosynostosis: a 12-year experience. Plast Reconstr Surg 2011;127(6):2397–406.

25. Utria AF, Mundinger GS, Bellamy JL, et al. The importance of timing in optimizing cranial vault remodeling in syndromic craniosynostosis. Plast Reconstr Surg 2015;135(4):1077–84.

26. de Jong T, Bannink N, Bredero-Boelhouwer HH, et al. Long-term functional outcome in 167 patients with syndromic craniosynostosis; defining a syndrome-specific risk profile. J Plast Reconstr Aesthet Surg 2010;63(10):1635–41.

27. Honnebier MB, Cabiling DS, Hetlinger M, et al. The natural history of patients treated for FGFR3-associated (Muenke-type) craniosynostosis. Plast Reconstr Surg 2008;121(3):919–31.

28. Wall SA, Goldin JH, Hockley AD, et al. Fronto-orbital re-operation in craniosynostosis. Br J Plast Surg 1994;47(3):180–4.

29. Levitt MR, Niazi TN, Hopper RA, et al. Resolution of syndromic craniosynostosis-associated Chiari malformation Type I without suboccipital decompression after posterior cranial vault release. J Neurosurg Pediatr 2012;9(2):111–5.

30. Spruijt B, Rijken BFM, den Ottelander BK, et al. First Vault Expansion in Apert and Crouzon-Pfeiffer Syndromes: Front or Back? Plast Reconstr Surg 2016; 137(1):112e–21e.

31. Nowinski D, Di Rocco F, Renier D, et al. Posterior cranial vault expansion in the treatment of craniosynostosis. Comparison of current techniques. Childs Nerv Syst 2012;28(9):1537–44.

32. Hersh DS, Hoover-Fong JE, Beck N, et al. Endoscopic surgery for patients with syndromic craniosynostosis and the requirement for additional open surgery. J Neurosurg Pediatr 2017;20(1):91–8.

33. Wenger TL, Hopper RA, Rosen A, et al. A genotype-specific surgical approach for patients with Pfeiffer syndrome due to W290C pathogenic variant in FGFR2 is associated with improved developmental outcomes and reduced mortality. Genet Med 2019;21(2):471–6.

34. Rottgers SA, Lohani S, Proctor MR. Outcomes of endoscopic suturectomy with postoperative helmet therapy in bilateral coronal craniosynostosis. J Neurosurg Pediatr 2016;18(3):281–6.

35. Rottgers SA, Syed HR, Jodeh DS, et al. Craniometric Analysis of Endoscopic Suturectomy for Bilateral Coronal Craniosynostosis. Plast Reconstr Surg 2019;143(1):183–96.

36. McCarthy JG, Glasberg SB, Cutting CB, et al. Twenty-year experience with early surgery for craniosynostosis: II. The craniofacial synostosis syndromes and pansynostosis–results and unsolved problems. Plast Reconstr Surg 1995;96(2):284–95. ; discussion 296-288.

37. Fearon JA. Beyond the bandeau: 4 variations on fronto-orbital advancements. J Craniofac Surg 2008;19(4):1180–2.

38. Adidharma W, Mercan E, Purnell C, et al. Evolution of Cranioorbital Shape in Nonsyndromic, Muenke, and Saethre-Chotzen Bilateral Coronal Synostosis: A Case-Control Study of 2-Year Outcomes. Plast Reconstr Surg 2021;147(1):148–59.

39. Ahmad F, Cobb ARM, Mills C, et al. Frontofacial monobloc distraction in the very young: a review of 12 consecutive cases. Plast Reconstr Surg 2012; 129(3):488e–97e.

40. Yang R, Shakoori P, Lanni MA, et al. Influence of Monobloc/Le Fort III Surgery on the Developing Posterior Maxillary Dentition and Its Resultant Effect on Orthognathic Surgery. Plast Reconstr Surg 2021; 147(2):253e–9e.

41. Bradley JP, Gabbay JS, Taub PJ, et al. Monobloc advancement by distraction osteogenesis decreases morbidity and relapse. Plast Reconstr Surg 2006;118(7):1585–97.

42. Arnaud E, Di Rocco F. Faciocraniosynostosis: monobloc frontofacial osteotomy replacing the two-stage strategy? Childs Nerv Syst 2012;28(9):1557–64.

43. Dunaway DJ, Britto JA, Abela C, et al. Complications of frontofacial advancement. Childs Nerv Syst 2012; 28(9):1571–6.

44. Dunaway DJ, Budden C, Ong J, et al. Monobloc Distraction and Facial Bipartition Distraction with External Devices. Clin Plast Surg 2021;48(3): 507–19.

45. Nassar AH, Mercan E, Massenburg BB, et al. Timing of Ossification of the Anterior Skull Base in Syndromic Synostosis. J Craniofac Surg 2020;31(5): 1256–60.

46. Hopper RA, Sandercoe G, Woo A, et al. Computed tomographic analysis of temporal maxillary stability and pterygomaxillary generate formation following pediatric Le Fort III distraction advancement. Plast Reconstr Surg 2010;126(5):1665–74.

47. Shetye PR, Boutros S, Grayson BH, et al. Midterm follow-up of midface distraction for syndromic craniosynostosis: a clinical and cephalometric study. Plast Reconstr Surg 2007;120(6):1621–32.

48. Goldstein JA, Paliga JT, Wink JD, et al. A craniometric analysis of posterior cranial vault distraction osteogenesis. Plast Reconstr Surg 2013;131(6):1367–75.

49. Swanson JW, Samra F, Bauder A, et al. An Algorithm for Managing Syndromic Craniosynostosis Using Posterior Vault Distraction Osteogenesis. Plast Reconstr Surg 2016;137(5):829e–41e.

50. Lauritzen C, Friede H, Elander A, et al. Dynamic cranioplasty for brachycephaly. Plast Reconstr Surg 1996;98(1):7–14. ; discussion 15-16.

51. Lauritzen CGK, Davis C, Ivarsson A, et al. The evolving role of springs in craniofacial surgery: the first 100 clinical cases. Plast Reconstr Surg 2008; 121(2):545–54.

52. Patel V, Shakir S, Yang R, et al. Perioperative Outcomes in the Treatment of Isolated Sagittal Synostosis: Cranial Vault Remodeling Versus Spring Mediated Cranioplasty. J Craniofac Surg 2020;31(7):2106–11.

53. White N, Evans M, Dover MS, et al. Posterior calvarial vault expansion using distraction osteogenesis. Childs Nerv Syst 2009;25(2):231–6.

54. Carlson AR, Taylor JA. Posterior vault distraction osteogenesis: indications and expectations. Childs Nerv Syst 2021;37(10):3119–25.

55. Derderian CA, Wink JD, McGrath JL, et al. Volumetric changes in cranial vault expansion: comparison of fronto-orbital advancement and posterior cranial vault distraction osteogenesis. Plast Reconstr Surg 2015;135(6):1665–72.

56. Humphries LS, Swanson JW, Bartlett SP, et al. Craniosynostosis: Posterior Cranial Vault Remodeling. Clin Plast Surg 2021;48(3):455–71.

57. Greives MR, Ware BW, Tian AG, et al. Complications in Posterior Cranial Vault Distraction. Ann Plast Surg 2016;76(2):211–5.

58. Abu-Sittah GS, Jeelani O, Dunaway D, et al. Raised intracranial pressure in Crouzon syndrome: incidence, causes, and management. J Neurosurg Pediatr 2016;17(4):469–75.

Syndromic Synostosis
Frontofacial Surgery

Kevin Chen, MD[a], Katelyn Kondra, MD[a], Eric Nagengast, MD, MPH[b],
Jeffrey A. Hammoudeh, MD, DDS[a,b,c,d,*], Mark M. Urata, MD, DDS[a,b,c,d]

KEYWORDS

- Syndromic craniosynostosis • Frontofacial surgery • Monobloc • Facial bipartition
- Orbital box osteotomies

KEY POINTS

- Frontofacial surgery can help treat the facial features of patients with syndromic craniosynostosis.
- Although monobloc/facial bipartition and orbital box osteotomies are complex and technically challenging procedures, they can be safely performed especially when done in conjunction with distraction.
- Patients with syndromic craniosynostosis are best managed by a multidisciplinary team.

Complex pediatric patients with genetic syndromes and craniosynostosis are most optimized by an interdisciplinary team of surgeons, pediatricians, geneticists, speech pathologists, audiologists, dietitians, pediatric dentists, orthodontists, and psychosocial support staff to manage the myriad of challenges and complications throughout early childhood and beyond. Despite early treatment of the anterior and posterior cranial vault, these patients frequently have resultant frontal and/or midface hypoplasia and orbital abnormalities that are best managed with simultaneous surgical treatment.

BACKGROUND AND HISTORY

Frontofacial surgery encompasses operations in which the orbits may be repositioned independently from or in conjunction with the maxilla and upper dental arch, namely, an orbital box osteotomy or a monobloc/bipartition, respectively. These powerful techniques allow a surgeon to correct orbitofacial disproportion with unilateral or bilateral orbital movements, to achieve orbitomaxillary segment advancement and correction of exorbitism. Beyond the aesthetic improvement with frontofacial surgery, operative intervention can improve functional respiratory status mitigating the need for tracheostomy, relieve intracranial pressure, improve occlusion and mastication, protect the corneas and globes, and enhance psychosocial interactions and maturity.

Frontofacial surgery has particular applicability for the patient with syndromic synostosis. Even if these patients have successful expansion of their cranial vault at an early age, many, if not all, have midface hypoplasia, hypertelorbitism, and exorbitism by the time they are entering school age.[1] As early as 1967, Tessier[2] published the need for total facial osteotomies to help treat patients with Apert and Crouzon syndromes. However, Ortiz-Monasterio[3] is ultimately credited with the development of the monobloc procedure as a method of simultaneous treatment of the cranial vault and midface in 1978. The very next year in 1979, Van der Meulen[4] expanded on the procedure by introducing

[a] Division of Plastic and Maxillofacial Surgery, Children's Hospital Los Angeles, 4650 West Sunset Boulevard, Mailstop 96, Los Angeles, CA 90027, USA; [b] Division of Plastic and Reconstructive Surgery, Keck Medicine of USC, 1520 San Pablo Street, Los Angeles, CA 90033, USA; [c] Herman Ostrow School of Dentistry, University of Southern California, 925 West 34th Street, Los Angeles, CA 90089, USA; [d] Division of Oral and Maxillofacial Surgery, University of Southern California, 925 West 34th Street, Los Angeles, CA 90089, USA
* Corresponding author. Division of Plastic and Maxillofacial Surgery, Children's Hospital Los Angeles, 4650 West Sunset Boulevard, Mailstop 96, Los Angeles, CA 90027.
E-mail address: jhammoudeh@chla.usc.edu

Oral Maxillofacial Surg Clin N Am 34 (2022) 459–466
https://doi.org/10.1016/j.coms.2022.03.001
1042-3699/22/© 2022 Elsevier Inc. All rights reserved.

the facial bipartition as a way to treat hypertelorism. Despite initial excitement, surgeons collectively revoked frontofacial advancement upon encountering major complications, such as cerebrospinal fluid (CSF) leaks, epidural abscesses, and frontal bone necrosis.[5] The historical narrative switched to preferential staging of the intracranial frontal advancement and the subsequent subcranial Le Fort III advancement.[6] It was not until distraction osteogenesis was applied to frontofacial procedures that they came back into relevancy.[7] The combination of monobloc/bipartition with distraction allowed for decreased complications as well as increased midface advancement, otherwise unachievable with single-stage advancement.

This article serves to highlight the aforementioned operations along with their indications and considerations while ultimately detailing their benefits to the complex facial skeleton of patients with syndromic craniosynostosis.

OPERATIVE TECHNIQUE
Monobloc

The operation is performed with the patient in the supine position on a horseshoe headrest. Bilateral tarsorrhaphies and a direct palatal splint are fabricated to protect the globes and teeth, respectively. A coronal incision is made from just superior to the root of the helix of the ear from one side of the scalp to the other. The incision is designed in a zigzag or stealth fashion to be less conspicuous in the hair line. Often, there is a pre-existing scar from an initial operation addressing the craniosynostosis. Dissection is carried anteriorly in the subperiosteal plane centrally to the superior orbital rims with care to protect the supraorbital neurovascular bundle. The

neurovascular bundle is released from the superior orbital foramen with a mallet and a small osteotome. In the midline, dissection is carried down to the nasal frontal junction. The periorbita is dissected free to expose all osteotomy sites. Laterally, the temporalis is left down, and the dissection plane is just superficial to the superficial layer of the deep temporal fascia. To approach the zygomatic arch, the dissection violates the superficial leaflet of the deep temporal fascia 1.5 cm above the arch; this allows entrance into the middle temporal fat pad. The zygomatic arch and body are exposed, and the dissection becomes confluent with the exposure of the frontal region. The temporalis may need to be partially freed from the bone at its most anterior aspect to achieve adequate exposure for the frontal craniotomy and expose the lateral orbital wall. Once the exposure is complete, the frontal craniotomy is marked by the craniofacial surgeon. **Fig. 1** demonstrates the coronal exposure. The superior aspect of the craniotomy should be at the height of contour of the calvarium to preserve shape of the skull after advancement; this is important because this segment will be advanced, so one does not want a "stair step," which can happen if one designs the posterior osteotomy too low. Once the frontal bone is removed, the frontal lobe and the anterior temporal lobe are dissected from the anterior cranial base to allow sufficient visualization and protection of the brain during the osteotomies. The authors' preference is to make the osteotomies with the Sonopet (Stryker; Kalamazoo, MI, USA), an ultrasonic osteotome. The first osteotomy performed is that of the lateral orbital wall. This osteotomy is performed with the ultrasonic knife externally through the lateral orbital wall starting at the lateral extent of the inferior orbital fissure (**Fig. 2**). While protecting the

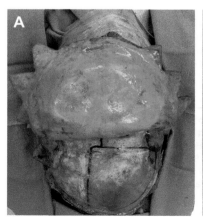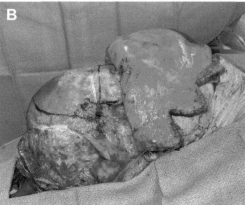

Fig. 1. Coronal exposure. (*A*) Axial view. (*B*) Lateral view.

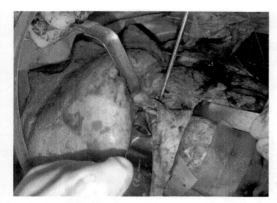

Fig. 2. Lateral wall osteotomy.

globe, the osteotomy continues superiorly and parallel to the lateral orbital rim and is continued simultaneously through the temporal bone laterally and the orbital roof centrally. A vertical osteotomy is then made through the zygomatic arch where the arch meets the body of the zygoma. The orbital floor osteotomy is then made. This osteotomy proceeds medially from the lateral aspect of the inferior orbital fissure parallel to the inferior orbital rim. Next, the orbital roof osteotomy is made. The osteotomy begins laterally at the previously performed roof osteotomy and proceeds parallel to the superior orbital rim and anterior to the cribriform plate. The medial orbital osteotomy is then completed from superior to inferior connecting to the previously performed medial orbital floor osteotomy. This osteotomy is parallel to the medial orbital rim and posterior to the medial canthus. The scalp flap is then placed back temporarily, and an intraoral upper vestibular incision is then made. A curved osteotome and mallet are used to complete pterygomaxillary separation. Rowe disimpaction forceps are placed in the nose externally or directly in the pyriform via the mouth. Slight downward traction is applied, and a long curved guarded osteotome is used to osteotomize the perpendicular plate of the ethmoid. The monobloc segment is then freed with the disimpaction forceps. The forceps are used in conjunction with laminar spreaders to mobilize the entire frontofacial complex. The monobloc can then be advanced directly and secured with plates at the frontal, temporal, and zygomatic arches or internal or external distractors can be applied. Our institution prefers to use internal distractors with accompanying C plates for vector control. A small 3-cm slit in the temporalis, parallel to the fibers and near the postauricular sulcus, is performed, and dissection is carried to the temporal bone bilaterally. The distractors are then situated such that

the anterior segment sits just superior to the zygomatic arch against the lateral orbital rim and parallel to the zygomatic arch. Care is taken to align bilateral distractors in a parallel vector. The distractor arm is then brought out to the postauricular skin through a stab incision, and the distractors are held in place with self-drilling/self-tapping screws. C plates are then placed in a class 3 configuration on the maxilla with a single central C plate on the anterior mandible; this allows vector control with use of different weights of orthodontic elastics.

Facial Bipartition

In a facial bipartition, the aforementioned steps are completed. Once the monobloc is downfractured, a central "V"-shaped portion can be marked for resection at the nasofrontal region. The inferior portion of the V is marked between the central incisors. The resection can be asymmetric if greater rotation is required for one side of the face compared with the other. During marking and bony resection, protection of the medial canthus is of utmost importance. Disruption of the medial canthus will lead to poor soft tissue movement and ultimately a worse outcome. The "V" resection is then cut from above using an ultrasonic osteotome. Then, from the intraoral incision, the maxilla and the hard palate are split in the midline again with the ultrasonic osteotome from the base of the pyriform aperture. The facial halves are then rotated superior-medially and fixated together at the midline frontal bone. The frontal sinuses are then cranialized. The frontal craniotomy bone is reshaped as needed and fixated to the bipartition segments. As with the monobloc, this construct can be advanced or distracted if necessary. **Fig. 3** demonstrates the postoperative scan of a patient undergoing bipartition surgery.

Orbital Box Osteotomies

In the box osteotomy, a similar approach is made. The osteotomies through the orbital walls are similar to those of the monobloc and facial bipartition. More posterior orbital osteotomies will allow for better repositioning of the globes after bony movement. In the box osteotomy procedure, pterygomaxillary disjunction is not necessary. Instead, through the gingivobuccal sulcus incision, the nasal mucosa is dissected free from the piriform, and the infraorbital nerves are identified. The inferior cut below the nerves of the "box" is made from the piriform directly laterally through the maxilla to connect with the lateral wall malar osteotomy. Medially, the planned resection of bone is marked.

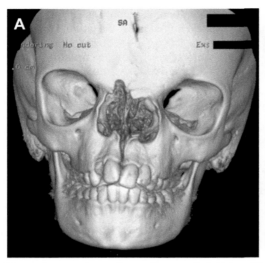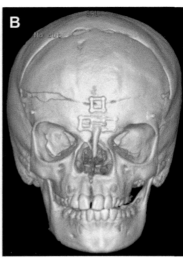

Fig. 3. 3D CT scan for a patient who underwent facial bipartition. (*A*) Preoperative scan. (*B*) Postoperative scan.

If there is a planned medial movement of the boxes, the transverse cuts of the box osteotomies need to be designed divergent toward the midline or with parallel cuts, otherwise the segments will not be able to move medially. Like in the bipartition, this resection does not need to be symmetric. Protection and preservation of the medial canthus is imperative. The medial box cuts are made from the top down intracranially with minimal dissection of the soft tissue off of the bone to preserve the canthus. The last described osteotomy is completed from above intracranially and is a continuation of the medial orbital wall osteotomy caudad through the lateral nasal wall to connect to the horizontal inferior box osteotomy that violates the pyriform. Once the orbital box is made, additional resections of bone may be made to rotate, raise, or lower the orbital complex. The orbital box osteotomy can be a unilateral or a bilateral procedure.

Virtual Surgical Planning and CAD/CAM

Virtual surgical planning can be extremely useful for helping to visualize the 3-dimensionality of the skull and even printing skull models to help plan and prebend the distractors; this can be useful especially for extremely asymmetric cases. The addition of cutting guides has not seemed to be helpful at the authors' institution because their decision making on the location of the bony cuts is largely performed intraoperatively after visualization of the full facial skeleton. The authors have not found a need for cutting guides that would justify the added cost because most osteotomies are performed using anatomic landmarks. In addition, the cutting guides do not assist with the

hardest cuts, which are the pterygomaxillary disjunction and the connection of the medial orbital wall osteotomy to the transverse osteotomy in the box osteotomy. Nonetheless, virtual surgical planning can be beneficial in certain circumstances especially if the surgeon is less experienced with frontofacial surgery.

INDICATIONS AND CONSIDERATIONS

Frontofacial surgery and its various techniques overlap in application to the syndromic patient, and depending on surgeon preference, multiple surgical approaches or various staged approaches can be used to treat similar orbital pathologies. However, there are important considerations for the selection of the surgical technique. The monobloc/bipartition can be performed at an earlier age than the orbital box osteotomy. The orbital box osteotomy necessitates a transverse maxillary cut, which obviously cannot be performed in mixed or primary dentition without sacrificing unerupted maxillary permanent teeth.

Early Intervention for Syndromic Patients

For some surgeons, patients with syndromic craniosynostosis are treated in a 2-stage fashion, with a fronto-orbital advancement before age 1 year and subsequent midface treatment later at age 5 to 6 years, or even later.[8,9] In general, this approach carries less risk of surgical morbidity than a single-stage approach with monobloc advancement. For the surgical algorithm, there must be flexibility and adaptation depending on the developing balance of the face. For patients who demonstrate frontofacial hypoplasia or hypertelorism, a monobloc or monobloc/facial bipartition with or without distraction may be the best comprehensive approach. In these cases, distraction of the monobloc complex will expand intracranial volume, advance the orbit to protect the globes and corneas, and advance the midface to improve airway obstruction, improve malocclusion, and potentially avoid tracheostomy or possibly lead to decannulation.

Destigmatization of the Syndromic Face

Regardless of the technique for treatment of the cranium, if the midface of a patient with syndromic craniosynostosis, such as Apert, Pfeiffer, or Crouzon, is left untreated, they generally develop facial stigmata as the facial skeleton continues to grow. These stigmata include orbital dystopia, most commonly in the horizontal plane with orbital hypertelorism, but can include an element of vertical orbital dystopia, and can also involve exotropia of the globes; downslanting palpebral fissures; and midface retrusion with a collapsed maxillary arch and inverted "V" deformity.[8,10] Patients who have more or all of these characteristics will have maximum benefit from monobloc with bipartition combined with distraction.

Monobloc with facial bipartition provides many benefits for the face of the syndromic patient. As described in the operative details prior, the bipartition procedure medializes the hemifacial segments by resecting a "V"-shaped segment of bone from the midline frontonasal region. When the remaining bony segments are brought together in the midline, the interdacryon distance is narrowed, the left orbit is rotated counterclockwise, and the right orbit is rotated clockwise. This rotation serves to improve the downward slanting palpebral fissures by elevating the entire lateral

canthal tendon and Whitnall tubercle complex. Rotating the entire complex improves the aesthetic balance of the medial to lateral palpebral fissures by elevating the lateral canthus above the medial canthus in a way that cannot be achieved by canthopexy or canthoplasty alone. In addition, rotating the orbits and bringing them closer together can improve the ophthalmologic exotropia.[11] When the hemifacial segments are brought together at the nasofrontal region, the segments rock against each other like seesaws and open at the maxilla, expanding the transverse width of the palate and improving the characteristic collapsed inverted "V" palate. **Figs. 4–6** demonstrate syndromic patients who have had improvement in facial balance after monobloc/bipartition.

As the bipartition segments are distracted forward, the midface retrusion improves, and exophthalmia is improved through advancement of the orbits relative to the globes. At the authors' institution, use of internal distractors is preferred because it is believed that there is less of a burden on the patients and their families, particularly in patients with Apert syndrome who have developmental delay. When the internal distractor is placed at the level of the zygoma, distraction of the monobloc/bipartition segments is mechanically advantageous over distraction of a Le Fort III segment. The distractor naturally sits at the center of the monobloc bony segment, allowing for a balanced anterior advancement, whereas it sits at the superiormost aspect of the Le Fort III bony segment, which will have a tendency to tip down as it advances anteriorly. Some centers argue for use of external distraction devices because these pull from the center of the face, improving collapse at the medial face, whereas internal distractors push from the lateral regions, potentially worsening collapse.[12] The authors have found that with rigid fixation of the medial bones at both the

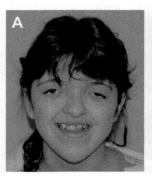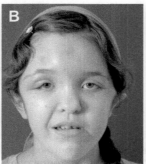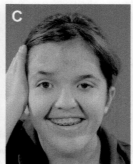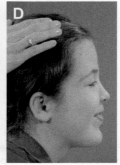

Fig. 4. Patient with Apert syndrome who underwent previous fronto-orbital advancement presenting for monobloc and facial bipartition distraction. (*A*) Preoperative photograph. (*B*) Three-month postoperative photograph. (*C*) Three-year postoperative frontal photograph. (*D*) Three-year postoperative lateral photograph.

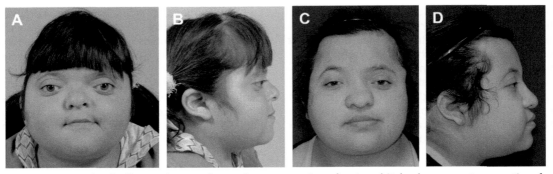

Fig. 5. Patient with Pfeiffer syndrome who underwent previous fronto-orbital advancement presenting for monobloc and facial bipartition without distraction. (*A*) Preoperative frontal photograph. (*B*) Preoperative lateral photograph. (*C*) Four-year postoperative frontal photograph. (*D*) Four-year postoperative lateral photograph.

frontal and anterior maxilla along with the use of C plates for multivector control, there is enough rigidity and flexibility to resist any collapse and successfully advance the monobloc/bipartition segments, which is corroborated by other institutions that regularly use internal distraction for these cases.[7,8,13]

Orbital Correction

If there is only midface hypoplasia, subcranial Le Fort III or III/I is a better option. Those patients,

on the other hand, with periorbital asymmetry or dystopia are best served by box osteotomies if the maxilla is in a good position. The flexibility of rotating the orbits independently or angling the infraorbital or supraorbital rims differentially is an underutilized tool from the authors' perspective. For the older patient in permanent dentition who requires treatment of orbital dystopia, horizontal or vertical, the orbital box osteotomy has become the preferred procedure. From a purely orbital positioning standpoint, the orbital box osteotomy

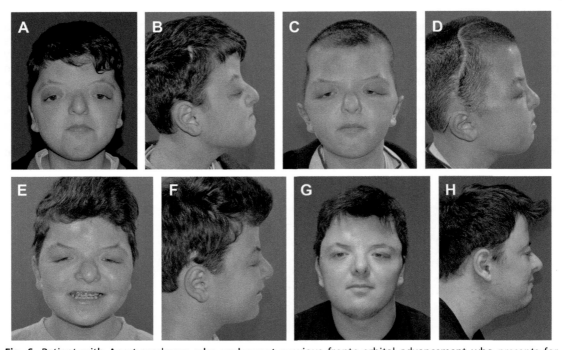

Fig. 6. Patient with Apert syndrome who underwent previous fronto-orbital advancement who presents for monobloc and facial bipartition with distraction. (*A*) Preoperative frontal photograph. (*B*) Preoperative lateral photograph. (*C*) Postoperative frontal photograph at the end of distraction. (*D*) Postoperative lateral photograph at the end of distraction. (*E*) One-year postoperative frontal photograph. (*F*) One-year postoperative lateral photograph. (*G*) Seven-year postoperative frontal photograph. (*H*) Seven-year postoperative lateral photograph.

offers many advantages over the facial bipartition. When performing the procedure, the medial wall cuts can be made without dissecting the medial canthus off of the nasal bone, preventing development of telecanthus and optimizing effect on the correction of hypertelorbitism. Many patients after facial bipartition can have a suboptimal result despite correction of the interdacryon distance because there is subtle stripping of the medial canthal tendon and as such, they develop some element of telecanthus even after resecuring the canthal tendons with wires.

After freeing the orbital box, the bony segment is able to move in more vectors than the hemifacial segment of a bipartition. To borrow terms from orthognathic surgery, freeing the orbital box allows for yaw, pitch, and roll of the segment, whereas the bipartition hemifacial segment is more or less restricted to roll. In particular, this is useful for yawing the segment and projecting the lateral orbital rim preferentially, an area that is frequently deficient in syndromic patients. For patients with asymmetric orbits, the 2 boxes can be moved in different vectors or even a unilateral orbital box osteotomy can be performed.

COMPLICATIONS

The complications and complication rate of frontofacial surgery have long been a topic of discussion given the need for intracranial exposure and osteotomy. When the monobloc procedure was introduced by Ortiz-Monasterio in 1978, surgeons were excited by such a powerful procedure that could simultaneously advance the frontal bone and orbital bandeau combined with the midface advancement of a Le Fort III segment.[3] Unfortunately, the large retrofrontal dead space led to intracranial infections that manifested as meningitis and epidural abscesses leading to bone loss, which quickly caused enthusiasm for the procedure to wane. Numerous papers at the time documented significantly higher infection rates when comparing Le Fort III to monobloc. Development of distraction osteogenesis and application to the monobloc procedure renewed its viability as a safe option that could generate significant facial change for syndromic patients. Bradley and colleagues[7] demonstrated that monobloc distraction had significantly fewer complications than traditional monobloc by minimizing initial retrofrontal dead space as well as allowing for remucosalization of the nasofrontal area before advancement, sealing off the nose from the brain.

Although some papers have reported that complication rates are still higher with monobloc advancement than Le Fort III advancement,[14] many institutions, including the authors', have found no significant difference in complication rates between the 2 procedures.[15,16] The authors also have found similar complication rates between monobloc distraction, monobloc distraction with facial bipartition, and facial bipartition alone.[13]

SUMMARY

Approaching the midface through an intracranial approach inherently increases the risks and morbidity of a procedure and introduces possibility for meningitis and CSF leaks. For the syndromic patient, frontofacial surgery, especially with distraction, has been proven to be safe and can be a transformative experience that can comprehensively improve their facial balance.

CLINICS CARE POINTS

- Monobloc with or without facial bipartition is a powerful procedure that can treat exorbitism, hypertelorism, midface hypoplasia, and frontal bone retrusion
- Orbital box osteotomies provide more flexibility for independent movement of the orbits in all directions
- Monobloc can be performed at an earlier age than orbital box osteotomies
- Patient selection is important because potential morbidity is more severe given intracranial approach; however, overall complication rate is comparable to subcranial procedures

FINANCIAL DISCLOSURE STATEMENT

The authors have no relevant financial interest to declare in relation to the content of this article.

REFERENCES

1. Kumar AR, Steinbacher D. Advances in the Treatment of Syndromic Midface Hypoplasia Using Monobloc and Facial Bipartition Distraction Osteogenesis. Semin Plast Surg 2014;28(4):179–83.
2. Tessier P. [Total facial osteotomy. Crouzon"s syndrome, Apert"s syndrome: oxycephaly, scaphocephaly, turricephaly]. Ann Chir Plast 1967;12(4):273–86.
3. Ortiz-Monasterio F, del Campo AF, Carrillo A. Advancement of the orbits and the midface in one piece, combined with frontal repositioning, for the correction of Crouzon's deformities. Plast Reconstr Surg 1978;61(4):507–16.

4. van der Meulen JC. Medial faciotomy. Br J Plast Surg 1979;32(4):339–42.

5. Wolfe SA, Morrison G, Page LK, et al. The monobloc frontofacial advancement: do the pluses outweigh the minuses? Plast Reconstr Surg 1993;91(6):977–87 [discussion: 988–9].

6. Fearon JA, Whitaker LA. Complications with facial advancement: a comparison between the Le Fort III and monobloc advancements. Plast Reconstr Surg 1993;91(6):990–5.

7. Bradley JP, Gabbay JS, Taub PJ, et al. Monobloc advancement by distraction osteogenesis decreases morbidity and relapse. Plast Reconstr Surg 2006;118(7):1585–97.

8. Raposo-Amaral CE, Vieira PH, Denadai R, et al. Treating syndromic craniosynostosis with monobloc facial bipartition and internal distractor devices. Clin Plast Surg 2021;48(3):521–9.

9. Paternoster G, Haber SE, Khonsari RH, et al. Craniosynostosis: Monobloc Distraction with Internal Device and Its Variant for Infants with Severe Syndromic Craniosynostosis. Clin Plast Surg 2021;48(3):497–506.

10. Raposo-Amaral CE, Denadai R, Ghizoni E, et al. Treating Craniofacial Dysostoses with Hypertelorism by Monobloc Facial Bipartition Distraction: Surgical and Educational Videos. Plast Reconstr Surg 2019;144(2):433–8.

11. Chen K, Duvvuri P, Bradley JP, et al. S13-02 Session 13: hypertelorism/craniofacial clefts improvement of exotropia in patients with hypertelorism corrected by facial bipartition. Plast Reconstr Surg Glob Open 2019;7. N2 - SN -(8S-2).

12. Greig AVH, Britto JA, Abela C, et al. Correcting the typical Apert face: combining bipartition with monobloc distraction. Plast Reconstr Surg 2013;131(2):219e–30e.

13. Goel P, Munabi NCO, Nagengast ES, et al. The Monobloc Distraction With Facial Bipartition: Outcomes of Simultaneous Multidimensional Facial Movement Compared With Monobloc Distraction or Facial Bipartition Alone. Ann Plast Surg 2020;84(5S Suppl 4):S288–94.

14. Zhang RS, Lin LO, Hoppe IC, et al. Retrospective review of the complication profile associated with 71 subcranial and transcranial midface distraction procedures at a single institution. Plast Reconstr Surg 2019;143(2):521–30.

15. Munabi NCO, Williams M, Nagengast ES, et al. Outcomes of intracranial versus subcranial approaches to the frontofacial skeleton. J Oral Maxillofacial Surg 2020;78(9):1609–16.

16. Meling TR, Høgevold H-E, Due-Tønnessen BJ, et al. Comparison of perioperative morbidity after LeFort III and monobloc distraction osteogenesis. Br J Oral Maxillofac Surg 2011;49(2):131–4.

Subcranial Midface Advancement in Patients with Syndromic Craniosynostosis

Benjamin B. Massenburg, MD[a,b], Srinivas M. Susarla, DMD, MD, MPH[a,b,c],
Hitesh P. Kapadia, DDS, PhD[b,d], Richard A. Hopper, MD, MS[a,b],*

KEYWORDS

- Subcranial surgery • Le Fort III Osteotomy • Le Fort II Osteotomy • Apert Syndrome
- Crouzon Syndrome • Pfeiffer Syndrome • Distraction Osteogenesis

KEY POINTS

- Midface morphology in patients with syndromic craniosynostosis is varied between the different types of syndromes.
- The midface in patients with Crouzon syndrome is more typically characterized by uniform hypoplasia, wherein there is congruent hypoplasia between the orbitozygomatic and nasomaxillary regions. These patients are effectively treated with Le Fort III advancement.
- The midface in patients with Apert/Pfeiffer syndromes is characterized by nasomaxillary hypoplasia that is more severe than orbitozygomatic hypoplasia. This population may benefit from segmental movements of the midface (eg, Le Fort II advancement with zygomatic repositioning).

INTRODUCTION

Craniosynostosis, or premature fusion of the cranial sutures, most commonly occurs in isolation, but it can also occur as part of a genetic syndrome with other associated anomalies. Patients with syndromic synostosis require comprehensive, multidisciplinary care from an experienced craniofacial team. Surgical interventions for these patients range from cranial vault expansion in infancy,[1] frontal or frontofacial surgery in childhood or adolescence,[2] subcranial midfacial advancement, to orthognathic surgery at skeletal maturity (**Fig. 1**).[3] Over the past 2 decades, there has been increased recognition of the distinct midface morphologies seen in the various syndromic craniosynostoses, with phenotype-specific protocols.[4–6]

The purpose of this article is to describe the approach to subcranial midface advancement for patients with syndromic synostosis. Subcranial surgery is typically performed in mixed dentition during early adolescence to correctly reposition (or overcorrect) the orbitozygomatic and nasomaxillary regions to restore developmental deficiencies. Midface advancement at this stage is focused on normalizing facial ratios and projection as well as expanding the pharynx to alleviate symptoms of airway obstruction. Recognition of the specific differences of each syndrome and patient by each anatomic region is critical for successful treatment. This article describes the unique facial phenotypes of common craniofacial syndromes, such as Apert, Pfeiffer, and Crouzon syndrome, and describes the surgical planning,

a Division of Plastic and Craniofacial Surgery, Seattle Children's Hospital, Craniofacial Center, Seattle, WA, USA; b Division of Plastic Surgery, Department of Surgery, University of Washington; c Department of Oral and Maxillofacial Surgery, University of Washington, Seattle, WA, USA; d Division of Craniofacial Orthodontics, Seattle Children's Hospital, Craniofacial Center, Seattle, WA, USA
* Corresponding author. Division of Plastic Surgery, Seattle Children's Hospital, 4800 Sand Point Way NE/ W7847, Seattle, WA 98105.
E-mail address: richard.hopper@seattlechildrens.org

Oral Maxillofacial Surg Clin N Am 34 (2022) 467–475
https://doi.org/10.1016/j.coms.2022.01.002
1042-3699/22/© 2022 Elsevier Inc. All rights reserved.

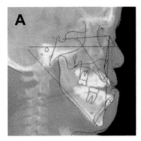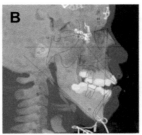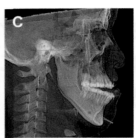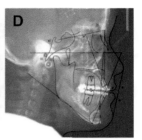

Fig. 1. Serial lateral cephalograms of a patient with Apert syndrome in the mixed dentition (*A*), after Le Fort II distraction with zygomatic repositioning (*B*), at skeletal maturity following orthodontic coordination (*C*), and following bimaxillary orthognathic surgery and genioplasty (*D*).

timing, operative execution of Le Fort III (LF3) or Le Fort II with zygomatic repositioning (LF2ZR), and postoperative care.

CLINICAL FINDINGS

The most common forms of syndromic synostosis are Apert, Crouzon, Pfeiffer, Muenke, and Saethre-Chotzen syndromes.[6] These most commonly present with bilateral coronal synostosis, midface hypoplasia, and possible extracranial deformities.

Apert syndrome occurs around 1 in 100,000 births owing to an autosomal dominant, gain-in-function mutation in the FGFR2 gene.[6] Midface hypoplasia in Apert syndrome is differentially distributed and has been called an "abnormal face in an abnormal position."[5,7] There is an axial as well as a sagittal concavity, which results in nasomaxillary deficiency

that is more severe than the orbitozygomatic deficiency (**Fig. 2**). Clinically, the orbitozygomatic deficiency is exhibited by poor malar support and exorbitism. The central midface demonstrates a severe vertical and sagittal deficiency,[8] exhibiting a class III skeletal relationship often with an anterior open bite.

Crouzon syndrome occurs around 1 in 65,000 births owing to an autosomal dominant with variable penetrance, gain-in-function mutation in the FGFR2 gene.[6] Midface hypoplasia in Crouzon syndrome is evenly distributed between the central and lateral midface and has been called a "normal face in an abnormal position" (**Fig. 3**).[5,7] Combined with relative mandibular prognathism, patients can present with severe class III skeletal relationships.

Pfeiffer syndrome occurs around 1 in 100,000 births owing to an autosomal dominant or

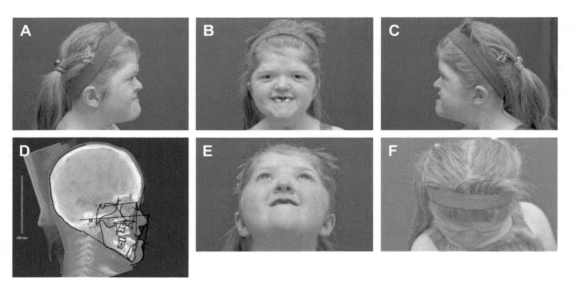

Fig. 2. Right lateral (*A*), anterior (*B*), left lateral (*C*), worm's eye (*E*), and top-down (*F*) images and lateral cephalogram (*D*) of a girl with Apert syndrome. She is exhibiting the characteristic midface hypoplasia (*A, C*), biconcavity phenotype with significantly more severe nasomaxillary deficiency than orbitozygomatic deficiency (*B, E, F*), and an anterior open bite (*B, D*).

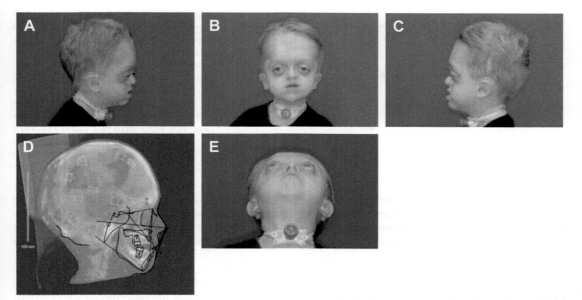

Fig. 3. Right lateral (*A*), anterior (*B*), left lateral (*C*), and worm's eye (*E*) images and lateral cephalogram (*D*) of a boy with Crouzon syndrome. He is exhibiting the characteristic congruent midface hypoplasia (*A, B, C, E*), and an anterior open bite (*A, B, C, D*).

sporadic gain-in-function mutation of FGFR2 (95%) or FGFR1 (5%). Midface hypoplasia in Pfeiffer syndrome is variable, with some patients presenting with evenly distributed hypoplasia similar to Crouzon syndrome and others presenting with a facial biconcavity similar to Apert syndrome.

Multidisciplinary care is mandatory throughout all stages of care for patients with syndromic synostosis. Regular ophthalmologic assessments are necessary for all patients with syndromic synostosis, as they are at risk for corneal exposure related to exorbitism, abnormalities in ocular motility, or intracranial hypertension. Patients undergoing these procedures are commonly in the mixed dentition, and dental and orthodontic evaluation and possible treatment must be performed before midface distraction.[9] In addition, airway and respiratory evaluation is essential to determine the severity of obstructive sleep apnea and the expected changes in sleep and breathing dynamics. In syndromic synostosis, the areas of obstruction are often multifocal,[10] and it is critical to understand the other tracheal or bronchial airway abnormalities impacting each patient.[11]

Treatment planning for correction of the midface deficiency seen in syndromic craniosynostosis requires a comprehensive dentofacial bony and soft tissue assessment, with particular attention to the cranial morphology, globe position, malar projection, nasal morphology, three-dimensional position of the maxilla and mandible, and occlusion.[9]

Three-dimensional computed tomographic scans are important for both diagnosis and surgical planning. They offer excellent visualization of the bony deficiencies as well as anatomic challenges like bony defects, shunts, nerves, or developing dentition (**Fig. 4**). Cast or digital models of the dentition are also essential for evaluating the premorbid occlusion, planning for the postoperative occlusion, identifying occlusal interferences, and fabricating splints.[9] Although surgical intervention to address the midface deficiency is best performed in the mixed dentition, it can be performed earlier if the child exhibits symptoms of severe obstructive sleep apnea or exorbitism. The benefits of earlier intervention need to be weighed against the risk of damage to the succedaneous maxillary dentition and need for repeat midface advancement in the setting of relapse. If the orbitozygomatic region is adequately advanced in early adolescence, the patient may only require traditional orthognathic surgery with Le Fort I and bilateral sagittal split osteotomies at skeletal maturity.[12] The goal for surgical management for patients with syndromic synostosis is to optimize the patient's form and function with the fewest interventions possible.

LE FORT III DISTRACTION

The LF3 osteotomy and advancement were pioneered by Gillies and Harrison[13] and later by Tessier[14] and has become a powerful tool to treat

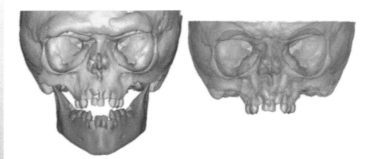

Fig. 4. Three-dimensional computed tomography scans of a patient with Apert syndrome with virtual surgical planning for the Le Fort II and III osteotomies and displaying the developing tooth buds to guide plate and screw placement. (*Adapted from* Susarla S, Hopper RA, Mercan E. Discussion: Airway Analysis in Apert Syndrome. Plast Reconstr Surg. 2019 Sep;144(3):710–712.)

midface hypoplasia, exorbitism with shallow orbits, malocclusion, obstructive sleep apnea, and facial imbalances. The development of distraction osteogenesis of the craniofacial skeleton by McCarthy and colleagues[15] was then applied to the LF3 osteotomy, and this offers decreased operative time and blood loss, the ability to perform larger advancements, no need for bone graft donor sites, and less relapse when compared with standard advancements.[16–18]

The exposure to the craniofacial skeleton for an LF3 osteotomy includes a zigzag, coronal incision that is elevated in the subperiosteal plane to the orbits and anterior zygomatic arch. The orbits should be degloved in a subperiosteal plane, in order to expose the lateral aspect of the inferior orbital fissure laterally and the posterior lacrimal crest and adjacent anterior ethmoid artery medially. To access the pterygomaxillary suture within the infratemporal fossa, the anterior aspect of the temporalis muscle is elevated, and dissection is carried subperiosteally behind the zygomatic body.

Once exposure is completed, a reciprocating saw should be used to perform the zygomatic arch osteotomy just behind the zygomatic body. This is followed by osteotomies from the junction of the frontozygomatic pillar to the inferior orbital fissure with a piezoelectric or reciprocating saw. An osteotome is used to continue the orbital floor osteotomy from the inferior orbital fissure to the uncinate process. Medially, a nasofrontal osteotomy is made with a piezoelectric saw, and this is continued to join the orbital floor osteotomy. The posterior maxillary sinus wall is the osteotomized down to the pterygomaxillary junction using a small osteotome placed through the orbital floor osteotomy. The pterygomaxillary separation can either be completed from this coronal approach or be completed intraorally. The final osteotomy is performed with a septal osteotome from the nasofrontal junction toward the posterior nasal spine, with special care taken to ensure the osteotomy remains anterior and inferior to the skull base,

particularly in patients with platybasia. Once all osteotomies have been made, the midface can be down-fractured carefully and mobilized to ensure that there are no interferences with the planned movement.

The primary distraction vector for LF3 advancement is anterior translation, which will expand the airway and improve the nasomaxillary and orbitozygomatic hypoplasia in parallel. The distraction vector can be angled inferiorly to lengthen the midface or nasal dorsum, or a clockwise rotation can be added to close an anterior open bite. Postoperatively, the end point of distraction is determined by the occlusion and the age of the patient, as there should be some overcorrection if the patient is not yet at skeletal maturity (**Fig. 5**).[19] Facial growth curves show completion of the upper midface growth around 8 years of age, with most of the remaining facial growth taking place in the mandible.[20,21]

LE FORT II WITH ZYGOMATIC REPOSITIONING

As previously discussed, the midface advancement achieved through LF3 distraction corrects exorbitism and malar hypoplasia through sagittal advancement of the inferior orbital rim and the body of the zygomas. However, this limits the sagittal advancement of the nasomaxillary region, as larger advancements will generate excessive orbital volume, and in the vertical dimension, as it will generate excessive orbital volume and height, increasing the risk for iatrogenic globe malposition. Thus, the central midface may be left undercorrected when trying to avoid enophthalmos in Apert syndrome. This specific morphologic, or an "abnormal face in an abnormal position," such as the phenotype found in Apert syndrome and some patients with Pfeiffer syndrome, can be addressed by using a segmental LF3 osteotomy, LF2ZR (**Fig. 6**), wherein there is differential movement of the central midface (via LF2 distraction) relative to the zygomas (via en bloc repositioning).[5,9]

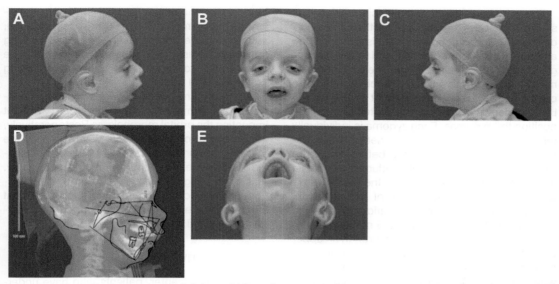

Fig. 5. Right lateral (*A*), anterior (*B*), left lateral (*C*), and worm's eye (*E*) images and lateral cephalogram (*D*) of the patient from **Fig. 3**, following LF3 distraction. The midface was advanced to an overcorrected position to account for the growing mandible, and he shows excellent lengthening of the nasal dorsum (*A, C*), malar and inferior orbital rim support (*B, E*), with a skeletal class II occlusion (*D*).

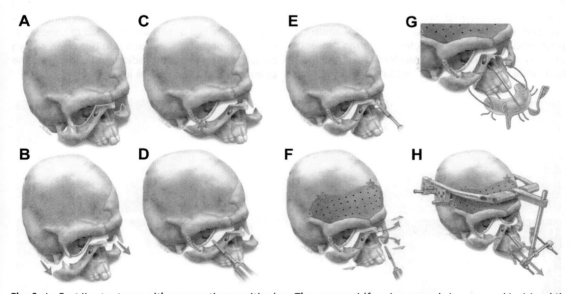

Fig. 6. Le Fort II osteotomy with zygomatic repositioning. The upper midface is accessed via a coronal incision (*A*). An LF3 osteotomy is performed, and the midface is downfractured (*B*). (*C*) The zygomatic bodies are then moved into an anterior and superior position (typically advanced 5–8 mm and impacted 3–5 mm and plated). Once this is completed, a Le Fort II osteotomy design is used to separate the nasomaxillary complex from the lateral orbito-zygomatic elements (*D–E*). The LF2 segment is then downfractured (*F*). A tooth-borne splint and external distraction device are then used to allow for an anterior and inferior movement of the central midface (*G, H*). Forehead deformities present at the time of subcranial surgery can be addressed simultaneously with a custom alloplastic cranial implant. (*From* Hopper RA, Kapadia H, Susarla SM. Le Fort II Distraction With Zygomatic Repositioning: A Technique for Differential Correction of Midface Hypoplasia. J Oral Maxillofac Surg. 2018 Sep;76(9):2002.e1-2002.e14; with permission.)

The exposure to the craniofacial skeleton is similar to that described above for the LF3 osteotomy and includes subperiosteal dissection of the anterior zygomatic arch, orbits, and nasofrontal regions from a coronal incision. The LF3 osteotomies, down-fracture, and mobilization are completed as described above. At this point, the LF3 segment is advanced and rotated to optimally position the zygomas. Each zygoma is individually repositioned and fixated, and then the hemi-Le Fort II osteotomy is performed before moving to the contralateral side. This reduces the strain across the midface and reduces the risk of maxillary fracture or displacement of prior fixation. Typical movements for zygomatic repositioning are 5 to 8 mm anterior and 3 to 5 mm superior.[22] The LF2 osteotomy is performed through an upper gingivobuccal sulcus incision using a piezoelectric saw, lateral to the infraorbital nerve. The coronal wound is then irrigated and closed with careful resuspension of the temporalis muscle.

A custom splint made with dental models or virtual surgical planning is then secured to the maxilla using 26-gauge steel wire loops through the piriform rim and lateral maxillary buttresses. Once the splint is secured, the intraoral incisions are irrigated and closed. Additional orthodontic bone anchors are placed at the midline of the maxilla and mandible. An external distraction device is then secured with cranial pins and a vertical midline post, and the transverse activation arms are set at a 30° to 45° downward vector from Frankfort horizontal. This distraction vector is determined by balancing the goals of increasing vertical maxillary height, correcting the maxillary occlusal plane, augmenting the dorsal nasal length, and leveling the palpebral fissures.[5] These activation arms are then secured to the maxillary traction splint using 24-gauge steel wires.

As the zygoma is already repositioned, the central LF2 segment can be distracted without impacting the orbital morphology. Postoperatively, the end point of distraction is determined by the maximal amount of advancement while maintaining medial eyelid contact without scleral show. This often brings the patient into an overjet position with associated mandibular hypoplasia that can be corrected with traditional orthognathic surgery at skeletal maturity (**Fig. 7**).

POSTOPERATIVE CARE

In the authors' center, patients who have undergone subcranial surgery are admitted to the intensive care unit and remain intubated for 2 to 3 days, until there is an air leak around the endotracheal tube. After a latency period of 3 to 5 days, distraction is begun at a rate of 1.0 to 1.5 mm per day. The shorter latency period and faster rate of distraction are used for younger patients, or more vertically oriented vectors, to prevent premature bony consolidation. After the desired movement is obtained, there is a 6- to 8-week period of consolidation, then once bony consolidate has been shown on lateral cephalogram radiographic imaging, the external distraction device is removed.

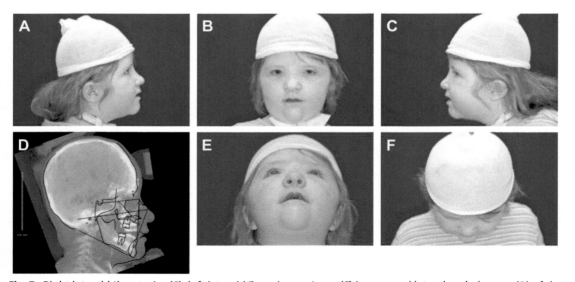

Fig. 7. Right lateral (*A*), anterior (*B*), left lateral (*C*), and worm's eye (*E*) images and lateral cephalogram (*D*) of the patient in **Fig. 2** following LF2ZR. There midface was advanced to an overcorrected position to account for the growing mandible. There is notable vertical lengthening of the central midface and nasal dorsum (*A, C*), as well as improved malar and inferior orbital rim support (*B, E, F*).

DISCUSSION

In appropriately selected patients, both LF3 and LF2ZR can be effective interventions to address midface hypoplasia, restore facial ratios, and improve obstructive sleep apnea. Morphometric analysis of facial ratios has demonstrated that patients with Apert syndrome have a midface-orbital height ratio that is significantly reduced when compared with normal controls, whereas patients with Crouzon syndrome have a facial ratio that is comparable to controls.[5] LF3 distraction moves the entire midface as a single unit, so the magnitude of anterior and inferior advancement is consistent across orbitale, anterior nasal spine, and A point.[5,23] In contrast, LF2ZR rigidly fixates the zygomas, allowing the central Le Fort II segment (nasomaxillary complex) to be independently distracted without impacting the orbital morphology. In LF2ZR, the A point and the anterior nasal spine can be inferiorly distracted, without any inferior translation of orbitale.[5,24] In a comparison of LF3 and LF2ZR in patients with Apert syndrome, LF2ZR was better able to correct the midface-orbital height ratio with independent, vertical central midface distraction.[5,24] The more vertical direction of the LF2ZR distraction vector results in a clockwise rotation of the palate, whereas the more horizontal distraction vector in LF3 results in a counterclockwise rotation of the palate.[25]

As the orbitozygomatic and nasomaxillary hypoplasia is uniform in Crouzon syndrome, LF3 distraction osteogenesis is the ideal subcranial surgery. With more severe nasomaxillary than orbitozygomatic hypoplasia in Apert syndrome and some cases of Pfeiffer syndrome, LF2ZR is ideal. Other segmental midfacial distraction procedures have been described, such as simultaneous, independent LF3 and Le Fort I advancement, in skeletally mature patients to separate the occlusal correction from the upper midface advancement,[26] using nasal passenger grafts[7] or cerclage hinges.[27]

Advancement of the midface following LF3 distraction has been shown to profoundly increase the volume of the nasopharyngeal airway, which can improve the symptoms of obstructive sleep apnea in a subset of patients with syndromic synostosis.[28–30] An evaluation of bony airway containing spaces following either LF3 or LF2ZR demonstrated that the volume of the nasopharynx increases by 54%, nasal airway increases by 35%, and oral airway increases by 16%.[25] This is consistent with data from other centers recognizing the nasopharyngeal airway as the site of maximal volumetric increase following midface

advancement.[30,31] The nasopharynx is one of the most common locations of obstruction for patients with syndromic synostosis, although it is often a multilevel problem with more than one anatomic area of obstruction.[10] In both LF3 and LF2ZR, the only distraction vector component to significantly impact the reduction of the apnea-hypopnea index (AHI) was the horizontal magnitude of distraction, reducing the AHI by 4.4 units for each 1 mm of horizontal movement.[25]

If the patient is simultaneously experiencing symptoms of increased intracranial pressure, a monobloc or facial bipartition procedure can simultaneously advance the midface and expand the anterior cranial vault.[2] Monobloc advances the LF3 segment, orbital bandeau, and frontal bone as one unit, whereas a bipartition can differentially advance the segments and allows more vector control if necessary.[32] Facial bipartition can narrow the facial width and correct the worms' eye concavity seen in Apert syndrome, but does not allow for vertical lengthening of the central midface or normalization of the oculofacial morphology.[33] These techniques will be described elsewhere in this issue of *Oral and Maxillofacial Surgery Clinics of North America* but do require an intracranial approach, which can increase the risk relative to isolated subcranial surgery.[34] In patients with forehead retrusion but no concern for elevated intracranial pressure, the authors place a custom forehead onlay implant at the time of device removal following an LF3 or LF2ZR.[22]

When considering transcranial versus subcranial interventions for management of midface deficiencies in syndromic craniosynostosis, the choice of intervention should be based on the individual patient morphology and symptoms.[34,35] The authors' protocol is to perform a posterior vault distraction early in infancy, followed by a fronto-orbital advancement (FOA) closer to 2 years of age, in recognition of the significant potential for relapse when the FOA is performed earlier in this population. A stable fronto-orbital correction in infancy may obviate frontofacial surgery and put the child on the path toward subcranial surgery in the mixed dentition and orthognathic surgery at skeletal maturity.[36] Although there are varied reports regarding whether transcranial interventions carry a significantly higher complication profile when compared with subcranial interventions, data from experienced centers have reported good results in appropriately selected patients.[34–37]

Complications occur in around 29% to 33% of patients undergoing subcranial surgery and are similar between both LF2ZR and LF3 distraction procedures.[24,34,35,38] Complications include infection, hardware malfunction, damage to the succedaneous maxillary dentition, unwanted fracture propagation resulting in intracranial injury, cerebrospinal fluid leaks from dural tears, incomplete advancement, and relapse.[34,35,38–40] Damage to the developing maxillary teeth can occur during the pterygomaxillary disjunction osteotomy or because of placing the screws of an internal distraction device into the tooth buds.[38,41] Overall complication rates are similar between internal and external distraction devices, but major infections requiring operating intervention may be more common with internal devices..[39] In this context, device selection is largely based upon surgeon and center experience. There have been reports of blindness or death following LF3 osteotomies, but these complications are notably rare in high-volume centers.[42]

SUMMARY

A clear understanding of the existing deformities and the expected changes that occur with surgery is fundamental to any reconstruction. The goals of LF3 distraction are to uniformly bring the infraorbital rims, zygomatic bodies, and nasomaxillary complex into optimal facial relationship, correcting congruent midface hypoplasia, restore facial ratios, and improve obstructive sleep apnea. The goals of Le Fort II distraction with zygomatic repositioning are to rigidly fixate the zygomas and lateral inferior orbital rims in the appropriate position, while further lengthening and advancing the central midface in patients with both sagittal and axial midfacial concavity, as seen in Apert or Pfeiffer syndrome. Timing of subcranial surgery is critical, and some overcorrection must be made before skeletal maturity to account for continued mandibular growth.

CLINICS CARE POINTS

- Patients with syndromic craniosynostosis undergoing subcranial midface osteotomies may have differing facial morphologies but share similarities insofar as management of medical comorbidities, such as obstructive sleep apnea.

- Following Le Fort II or Le Fort III osteotomies for subcranial distraction, patients are admitted to the intensive care unit and remain intubated and sedated for 2 to 3 days, until there is an air leak around the endotracheal tube.

- After a latency period of 3 to 5 days, distraction is begun at a rate of 1.0 to 1.5 mm per day.

- Once the desired subcranial advancement is obtained, there is a 6- to 8-week period of consolidation.

- After bony generate is evident on imaging, the external distraction device is removed.

REFERENCES

1. Shakir S, Birgfeld CB. Syndromic synostosis: cranial vault expansion in infancy. Oral Maxillofac Surg Clin 2022.
2. Hammoudeh JA, Urata MM. Syndromic synostosis: frontofacial surgery. Oral Maxillofac Surg Clin 2022.
3. Han J, Egbert MA, Ettinger RE, et al. Orthognathic surgery in patients with syndromic synostosis. Oral Maxillofac Surg Clin 2022.
4. Taylor JA, Bartlett SP. What's new in syndromic craniosynostosis surgery? Plast Reconstr Surg 2017; 140(1):82e–93e.
5. Hopper RA, Kapadia H, Morton T. Normalizing facial ratios in apert syndrome patients with Le Fort II midface distraction and simultaneous zygomatic repositioning. Plast Reconstr Surg 2013;132(1):129–40.
6. Forrest CR, Hopper RA. Craniofacial syndromes and surgery. Plast Reconstr Surg 2013;131(1):86–109.
7. Hopper RA, Prucz RB, Iamphongsai S. Achieving differential facial changes with Le Fort III distraction osteogenesis: the use of nasal passenger grafts, cerclage hinges, and segmental movements. Plast Reconstr Surg 2012;130(6):1281–8.
8. Oberoi S, Hoffman WY, Vargervik K. Craniofacial team management in Apert syndrome. Am J Orthod Dentofacial Orthop 2012;141(4 suppl):S82–7.
9. Hopper RA, Kapadia H, Susarla SM. Surgical-orthodontic considerations in subcranial and frontofacial distraction. Oral Maxillofac Surg Clin N Am 2020; 32(2):309–20.
10. Doerga PN, Spruijt B, Mathijssen IMJ, et al. Upper airway endoscopy to optimize obstructive sleep apnea treatment in Apert and Crouzon syndromes. J Cranio-Maxillofacial Surg 2016;44(2):191–6.
11. Wenger TL, Hopper RA, Rosen A, et al. A genotype-specific surgical approach for patients with Pfeiffer syndrome due to W290C pathogenic variant in FGFR2 is associated with improved developmental outcomes and reduced mortality. Genet Med 2019; 21(2):471–6.
12. Warren SM, Shetye PR, Obaid SI, et al. Long-term evaluation of midface position after Le Fort III advancement: a 20-plus-year follow-up. Plast Reconstr Surg 2012;129(1):234–42.
13. Gillies SH, Harrison SH. Operative correction by osteotomy of recessed malar maxillary compound in a case of oxycephaly. Br J Plast Surg 1950;3(C): 123–7.

14. Tessier P. Total osteotomy of the middle third of the face for faciostenosis or for sequelae of Le Fort III fractures. Plast Reconstr Surg 1971;48(6):533–41.

15. McCarthy JG, Schreiber J, Karp N, et al. Lengthening the human mandible by gradual distraction. Plast Reconstr Surg 1992;89(1):1–8.

16. Saltaji H, Altalibi M, Major MP, et al. Le Fort III distraction osteogenesis versus conventional Le Fort III osteotomy in correction of syndromic midfacial hypoplasia: a systematic review. J Oral Maxillofac Surg 2014;72(5):959–72.

17. Hopper RA, Ettinger RE, Purnell CA, et al. Thirty years later: what has craniofacial distraction osteogenesis surgery replaced? Plast Reconstr Surg 2020;145(6):1073e–88e.

18. Fearon JA. Le Fort III osteotomy or distraction osteogenesis imperfecta. Plast Reconstr Surg 2007; 119(3):1122–3.

19. Patel N, Fearon JA. Treatment of the syndromic midface: a long-term assessment at skeletal maturity. Plast Reconstr Surg 2015;135(4):731e–42e.

20. Buschang PH, Baume RM, Nass GG. A craniofacial growth maturity gradient for males and females between 4 and 16 years of age. Am J Phys Anthropol 1983;61(3):373–81.

21. Ranly DM. Craniofacial growth. Dent Clin North Am 2000;44(3):457–470, v.

22. Hopper RA, Wang HD, Mercan E. Le Fort II distraction with simultaneous zygomatic repositioning. Clin Plast Surg 2021;48(3):487–96.

23. Shetye PR, Davidson EH, Sorkin M, et al. Evaluation of three surgical techniques for advancement of the midface in growing children with syndromic craniosynostosis. Plast Reconstr Surg 2010;126(3):982–94.

24. Purnell CA, Evans M, Massenburg BB, et al. Lefort II distraction with zygomatic repositioning versus Lefort III distraction: A comparison of surgical outcomes and complications. J Cranio-Maxillofacial Surg. 2021;56(1):61.

25. Liu MT, Kurnik NM, Mercan E, et al. Magnitude of horizontal advancement is associated with apnea hypopnea index improvement and counterclockwise maxillary rotation after subcranial distraction for syndromic synostosis. J Oral Maxillofac Surg 2021;79(5):1133.e1-6.

26. Hammoudeh JA, Goel P, Wolfswinkel EM, et al. Simultaneous midface advancement and orthognathic surgery: a powerful technique for managing midface hypoplasia and malocclusion. Plast Reconstr Surg 2020;145(6):1067e–72e.

27. Denny AD, Kalantarian B, Hanson PR. Rotation advancement of the midface by distraction osteogenesis. Plast Reconstr Surg 2003;111(6):1789–99.

28. Flores RL, Shetye PR, Zeitler D, et al. Airway changes following Le Fort III distraction osteogenesis for syndromic craniosynostosis: a clinical and cephalometric study. Plast Reconstr Surg 2009;124(2):590–601.

29. Ettinger RE, Hopper RA, Sandercoe G, et al. Quantitative computed tomographic scan and polysomnographic analysis of patients with syndromic midface hypoplasia before and after Le Fort III distraction advancement. Plast Reconstr Surg 2011;127(4):1612–9.

30. Nout E, Bouw FP, Veenland JF, et al. Three-dimensional airway changes after Le Fort III advancement in syndromic craniosynostosis patients. Plast Reconstr Surg 2010;126(2):564–71.

31. Xu H, Yu Z, Mu X. The assessment of midface distraction osteogenesis in treatment of upper airway obstruction. J Craniofac Surg 2009;20(8 SUPPL. 2):1876–81.

32. Ponniah AJT, Witherow H, Richards R, et al. Three-dimensional image analysis of facial skeletal changes after monobloc and bipartition distraction. Plast Reconstr Surg 2008;122(1):225–31.

33. Glass GE, Ruff CF, Crombag GAJC, et al. The role of bipartition distraction in the treatment of apert syndrome. Plast Reconstr Surg 2018;141(3):747–50.

34. Zhang RS, Lin LO, Hoppe IC, et al. Retrospective review of the complication profile associated with 71 subcranial and transcranial midface distraction procedures at a single institution. Plast Reconstr Surg 2019;143(2):521–30.

35. Munabi NCO, Williams M, Nagengast ES, et al. Outcomes of intracranial versus subcranial approaches to the frontofacial skeleton. J Oral Maxillofac Surg 2020;78(9):1609–16.

36. Hopper RA. Discussion: retrospective review of the complication profile associated with 71 subcranial and transcranial midface distraction procedures at a single institution. Plast Reconstr Surg 2019; 143(2):531–2.

37. Dunaway DJ, Britto JA, Abela C, et al. Complications of frontofacial advancement. Child's Nerv Syst 2012; 28(9):1571–6.

38. Fearon JA. Halo distraction of the Le Fort III in syndromic craniosynostosis: a long-term assessment. Plast Reconstr Surg 2005;115(6):1524–36.

39. Goldstein JA, Thomas Paliga J, Taylor JA, et al. Complications in 54 frontofacial distraction procedures in patients with syndromic craniosynostosis. J Craniofac Surg 2015;26(1):124–8.

40. Greig AVH, Davidson EH, Grayson BH, et al. Complications of craniofacial midface distraction: 10-year review. Plast Reconstr Surg 2012;130(2):371–2.

41. Sicard L, Hounkpevi M, Tomat C, et al. Dental consequences of pterygomaxillary dysjunction during fronto-facial monobloc advancement with internal distraction for Crouzon syndrome. J Cranio-Maxillofacial Surg. 2018;46(9):1476–9.

42. Czerwinski M, Hopper RA, Gruss J, et al. Major morbidity and mortality rates in craniofacial surgery: an analysis of 8101 major procedures. Plast Reconstr Surg 2010;126(1):181–6.

Orthognathic Surgery in Patients with Syndromic Craniosynostosis

Jesse T. Han, DDS, MD[a], Mark A. Egbert, DDS[a,b,c], Russell E. Ettinger, MD[b,c], Hitesh P. Kapadia, DDS, PhD[b,c], Srinivas M. Susarla, DMD, MD, MPH[a,b,c,*]

KEYWORDS

- Craniosynostosis • Midface deficiency • Maxillary hypoplasia • Orthognathic surgery
- Le Fort I osteotomy • Sagittal split osteotomy • Apert syndrome • Crouzon syndrome

KEY POINTS

- Patients with syndromic craniosynostosis may have undergone subcranial midface advancement, typically via distraction osteogenesis, in the mixed dentition. Performing a Le Fort I osteotomy at skeletal maturity in these patients requires an understanding of the effects of subcranial distraction on the maxilla.
- The end-stage skeletal discrepancy in patients with syndromic craniosynostosis is related primarily to residual midface deficiency at the Le Fort I level, but may also involve some degree of mandibular deformity. Bimaxillary surgery is frequently required to fully address the maxillomandibular discrepancy.
- Residual upper airway obstruction may be present even after subcranial midface distraction and remains an important consideration in treatment planning.
- Patients with nonsyndromic craniosynostosis may also present with maxillomandibular discrepancies, such as facial scoliosis seen in patients with unilateral coronal synostosis.

INTRODUCTION

Craniosynostosis results from premature fusion of a cranial vault suture, inhibiting normal skull growth perpendicular to the fused suture, with compensatory growth parallel to the fused suture. Overall, craniosynostosis occurs in 1:2000 to 1:2500 births; craniosynostosis syndromes occur in 1:25,000 to 1:100,000 births.[1,2] The most common syndromes associated with craniosynostosis are Apert, Carpenter, Crouzon, Pfeiffer and Saethre–Chotzen syndromes. Advances in genetic diagnostics have revealed fibroblast growth factor receptor (FGFR), and TWIST mutations as the most common causes of craniosynostosis syndromes.

While patients with syndromic craniosynostosis may initially present with abnormalities in cranial vault and fronto-orbital morphology, the cranial base and midface sutures are affected as well, frequently resulting in midface hypoplasia.[3] The spheno-occipital synchondrosis is one of the last synchondroses of the cranial base to fuse and its premature fusion in craniosynostosis is hypothesized to be a cause of midface hypoplasia.[4] Growth restriction in the midface leads to stereotypical dysmorphologies including exorbitism, deficiency in nasal length, maxillary retrusion, a high-arched palate, and dental crowding.

Operative management of syndromic synostosis takes into consideration the presence of

[a] Department of Oral and Maxillofacial Surgery, University of Washington School of Dentistry, Seattle, WA, USA; [b] Department of Surgery, Division of Plastic Surgery, University of Washington School of Medicine, Seattle, WA, USA; [c] Craniofacial Center, Seattle Children's Hospital, Seattle, WA, USA
* Corresponding author. Craniofacial Center, Seattle Children's Hospital, 4800 Sand Point Way NE, Seattle, WA 98105.
E-mail address: SRINIVAS.SUSARLA@SEATTLECHILDRENS.ORG

increased intracranial pressure (ICP), airway obstruction, and facial dysmorphology. While early interventions during active growth are aimed at addressing cephalocranial disproportion (eg, posterior vault distraction and fronto-orbital advancement in infancy) and upper midface dysmorphology (eg, Le Fort II or Le Fort III osteotomies in the mixed dentition), orthognathic surgery is typically reserved to correct remaining dentofacial deformities when skeletal maturity is achieved (**Fig. 1**). The purpose of this article is to review the anatomic and operative considerations for patients with craniosynostosis as they relate to the correction of end-stage skeletal discrepancies using orthognathic surgery.

ANATOMIC CONSIDERATIONS

Maxilla: Once thought to be related to premature fusion of the major calvarial sutures, midface deficiency in syndromic synostosis (**Fig. 2**) is now understood to result from premature fusion of cranial base suture. In 1986, Burdi and colleagues hypothesized that premature closure of the spheno-ethmoidal synchondrosis prevented normal maxillary development.[4] Premature closure of the spheno-occipital synchondrosis has been more recently studied as another source of midface deficiency. When compared with matched controls,

the spheno-occipital synchondrosis was closed significantly earlier in patients with Apert syndrome.[5] The circum-maxillary sutures are also under investigation as a contributing cause of midface deficiency.[6] While primarily studied in the context of syndromic craniosynostosis, there is evidence suggesting that patients with unilateral coronal synostosis may share similar pathology underlying the development of facial scoliosis (**Fig. 3**).[7]

Clinically, the midface deficiency in syndromic synostosis occurs in multiple dimensions. Forte and colleagues found that the average maxillary anteroposterior (AP) length in previously untreated Apert and Crouzon patients was significantly shorter at 4.39 ± 0.49 cm, compared to 4.96 ± 0.46 cm in matched controls, resulting in a Class III malocclusion.[8] Abnormal maxillary development also results in transverse growth restriction. These authors also reported that the average maxillary width in untreated Apert and Crouzon patients in their study was 6.23 ± 0.85 cm and 5.71 ± 0.63 cm, respectively. There is notable variability in the characteristics of the midface dysmorphology seen in patients with Crouzon syndrome relative to those with Apert/Pfeiffer syndrome (see **Fig. 2**A,B). Patients in the latter diagnostic group tend to have more severe nasomaxillary hypoplasia relative to

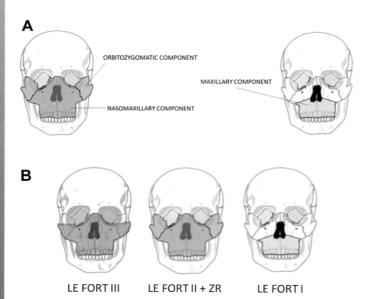

A

ORBITOZYGOMATIC COMPONENT

MAXILLARY COMPONENT

NASOMAXILLARY COMPONENT

B

LE FORT III   LE FORT II + ZR   LE FORT I

Fig. 1. (*A*) The maxillofacial skeletal discrepancy seen in patients with syndromic craniosynostosis will primarily involve the midface. The midface components can be divided into the orbitozygomatic and nasomaxillary components; the nasomaxillary region can be further subdivided into a maxillary component and a nasal component. (*B*) Osteotomy choice for the correction of midface hypoplasia is dependent upon the highest level affected. In patients with uniform midface hypoplasia, where the orbitozygomatic hypoplasia is congruent with the nasomaxillary hypoplasia, a Le Fort III osteotomy in the mixed dentition may be indicated to advance the midface to address the malar deficiency and exorbitism. In patients whereby the central midface hypoplasia is more severe than the lateral midface hypoplasia, segmental movements of the midface via Le Fort II osteotomy with en bloc zygomatic repositioning (ZR) may be indicated to allow anterior and inferior distraction of the nasomaxillary complex and independent anterior–superior repositioning of the zygoma to address the malar hypoplasia and exorbitism. At skeletal maturity, nearly all patients with syndromic craniosynostosis will have midface hypoplasia affecting the lower midface. Le Fort I osteotomy is indicated in these patients to address the lower midface hypoplasia and occlusion. (*Adapted from* Hopper RA, Kapadia H, Susarla SM. Surgical-Orthodontic Considerations in Subcranial and Frontofacial Distraction. Oral Maxillofac Surg Clin North Am. 2020 May;32(2):309-320.)

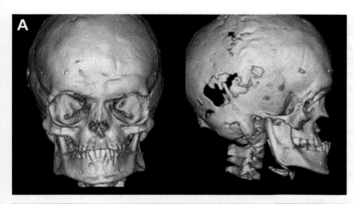

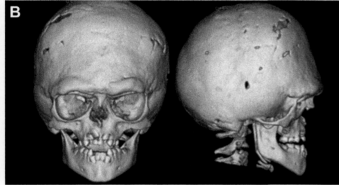

Fig. 2. In patients with Crouzon syndrome, there is global midface hypoplasia wherein the nasomaxillary hypoplasia and orbitozygomatic hypoplasia are congruent (A). These patients may benefit from Le Fort III distraction in the mixed dentition. () In contrast, patients with Apert/Pfeiffer syndrome will have nasomaxillary hypoplasia that is more severe than orbitozygomatic hypoplasia (B) and may benefit from segmental subcranial midface advancement (Le Fort II + zygomatic repositioning) in the mixed dentition. The maxillary component of the midface hypoplasia is best addressed at skeletal maturity via Le Fort I osteotomy, which will effectively address both the three-dimensional skeletal dysmorphology and occlusion. (Adapted from Hopper RA, Kapadia H, Susarla SM. Surgical-Orthodontic Considerations in Subcranial and Frontofacial Distraction. Oral Maxillofac Surg Clin North Am. 2020 May;32(2):309-320.)

orbitozygomatic hypoplasia and may benefit from segmental midface movements in the mixed dentition.

Mandible: Like the maxilla, mandibular growth is also altered in patients with syndromic synostosis. One hypothesis of altered mandibular development is that midface deficiency causes mandibular autorotation.[9] Another hypothesis is that intrinsic FGFR mutations alter mandibular morphology. *In vivo* studies in mice have revealed that FGFR mutations result in decreased bone volume and development.[10] These mutations also result in decreased bone content of calcium and phosphate thought to be due to changes in osteoblast and osteoclast physiology.

Altered mandibular development results in numerous characteristic mandibular findings in syndromic synostosis. Kreiborg studied 55 patients with different types of syndromic synostosis and concluded that the affected mandible is similar in size to nonsyndromic patients but that a relative downward tilt of the maxilla creates a

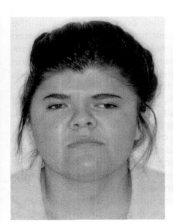

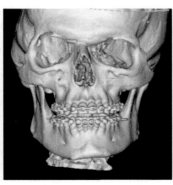

Fig. 3. This patient with unilateral coronal craniosynostosis underwent fronto-orbital advancement in infancy. At skeletal maturity, she has nasal and maxillomandibular asymmetry (facial twist), with associated malocclusion. Bimaxillary orthognathic surgery with rotation of the maxillomandibular complex in the coronal plane, as well as a rhinoseptoplasty, is indicated for correction of the end-stage facial skeletal difference.

"wedge effect" of the mandible resulting in a high mandibular plane angle, apertognathia and relative prognathism.[11] Costaras-Volarich and Pruzansky measured mandibular dimensions of patients with Apert and Crouzon syndromes and found the mandibular ramus was longer and the body was shorter in these patients than controls, creating an L-shaped mandible.[12] Three-dimensional analysis of mandibular morphology in patients with Apert syndrome demonstrated that, while there was no difference in mandibular volume compared with controls, the Apert group had shorter mandibular lengths.[13]

Dentoalveolar morphology: Dental arch morphology is also influenced by multi-suture synostosis. The altered development of the maxilla and mandible is thought to decrease dental arch dimensions resulting in high arched palates, narrow maxillary dental arches, dental crowding, and malocclusion (**Fig. 4**). A longitudinal study by Reitsma and colleagues found that patients with Apert and Crouzon syndrome had significantly smaller dental arches compared with control patients.[14] This study also found that patients with Apert and Crouzon syndrome had a higher prevalence of dental agenesis, which is thought to also decrease the growth potential of the dental arch. A retrospective chart review by Agochukwu and colleagues of 21 patients with Muenke syndrome found that 67% had a high arched palate.[15] Mandibular arch length was also found to be significantly smaller in patients with syndromic synostosis compared with controls.[14]

TREATMENT CONSIDERATIONS

Presurgical orthodontic treatment: Well before reaching skeletal maturity, patients with syndromic synostosis should be evaluated for the need for orthognathic surgery by a multi-disciplinary team consisting of orthodontists, pediatric dentists, and surgeons. Patients should have regular dental examinations in preparation for orthodontics. In the mixed-dentition phase, particular attention should be paid toward expanding and leveling the maxillary arch. Caution should be exercised when planning a palatal expansion for patients with synostosis, as circum-maxillary sutures may be fused and attempt to widen the maxillary arch in these patients may cause damage to deciduous teeth. The surgeon and orthodontist should work together to determine whether extraction therapy is indicated to correct the arch length discrepancies. Planning for final arch coordination begins in the mixed dentition.

Patients with syndromic synostosis should also be assessed for obstructive sleep apnea during this time period. Many patients may undergo subcranial midface advancement at this stage to address the upper midface morphology and also afford some degree of upper airway expansion. The selection of upper midface osteotomy design is predicated primarily on the degree of hypoplasia of both the orbitozygomatic and nasomaxillary components of the midface. In patients whereby it is congruent, global midface hypoplasia (eg, Crouzon syndrome), Le Fort III distraction may be the procedure of choice. In patients with

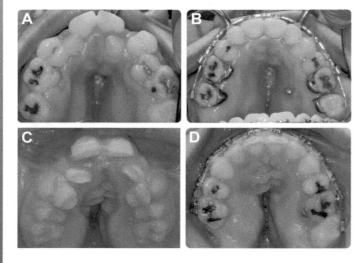

Fig. 4. Patients with syndromic craniosynostosis will frequently present with constricted maxillary arch forms characterized by high arched palates, narrow maxillary dental arches, dental crowding, oligodontia, and malocclusion. Coordinated treatment planning for the final occlusion begins in the mixed dentition and requires shared decision-making between the orthodontist and surgeon. The maxillary arch form in a patient with Crouzon syndrome is seen in the mixed dentition before orthodontic treatment (*A*) and at the end of presurgical orthodontic treatment, including palatal expansion, in the anticipation of orthognathic surgery (*B*). Similar dentoalveolar morphology can be seen in patients with Apert syndrome: (*C*) mixed dentition before orthodontic treatment, and (*D*) following orthodontic coordination, including palatal expansion and premolar extractions, in preparation for orthognathic surgery.

primary nasomaxillary hypoplasia, Le Fort II distraction may be a more suitable option. Patients with nonuniform midface hypoplasia (eg, Apert and Pfeiffer syndromes), wherein the nasomaxillary hypoplasia is more severe than the orbitozygomatic hypoplasia, may benefit from segmental movements such as Le Fort II distraction with zygomatic repositioning.[16–20]

Orthognathic surgery: Orthognathic surgery in this population has been found to be safe, in general.[21–23] A retrospective chart review conducted on 8340 subjects admitted postoperatively after orthognathic surgery with various craniofacial anomalies found an overall complication rate of 9.1%.[21] This rate is similar to a review of postoperative complications following orthognathic surgery in an otherwise normal population of 1294 subjects, which showed a 9.7% complication rate.[21] The most common complications were bacterial infection (2.4%), hemorrhage (2.0%) and postoperative pneumonia (1.8%). The study found that 95% of the subjects were routinely discharged after a median hospital admission length of 1.7 days.

Outcomes of orthognathic surgery also show good results in the syndromic synostosis population. A retrospective review of patients with syndromic and nonsyndromic synostosis found that, of the 39 subjects who underwent orthognathic surgical correction of end-stage skeletal discrepancies, 4 had relapse.[23]

Maxillary surgery: Given the complex maxillary morpholology in patients with syndromic synostosis, treatment planning for maxillary osteotomies can be challenging. As mentioned previously, the maxilla in these patients has deficiencies in the multiple dimensions and will often require advancement as well as occlusal plane alterations to close anterior open bites. Most patients will present with some degree of maxillary sagittal hypoplasia, necessitating advancement at the Le Fort I level. Ideal maxillary sagittal positioning can be achieved based on linear or angular measurements, but the surgeon should consider the forehead morphology, which may be altered due to prior fronto-orbital advancement and cranioplasty when using methodologies such as Andrews' analysis.[24] Occlusal plane alterations are frequently necessary to address the vertical position of the maxilla and an anterior open bite and can include posterior–superior repositioning of the maxilla, anterior inferior repositioning of the maxilla, counterclockwise rotation of the mandible, or a combination of these movements (**Fig. 5**). Segmental osteotomies may be necessary to correct persistent transverse defects or adjust biplanar occlusions.

Maxillary osteotomies in previously distracted patients: Le Fort I osteotomies in these patients can be made more challenging when accompanied by a history of cleft palate or the multiply

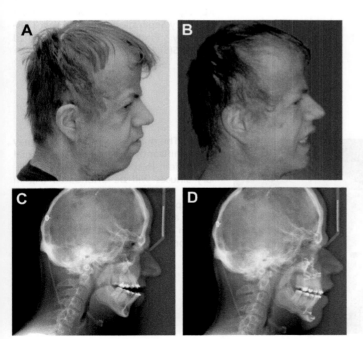

Fig. 5. This patient with Crouzon syndrome was treated with a Le Fort III subcranial distraction in the mixed dentition. At skeletal maturity, he has an end-stage deformity characterized by posterior vertical maxillary excess, anterior vertical maxillary hypoplasia, maxillary sagittal hypoplasia, and a large anterior open bite (*A, B*). He was successfully treated with a Le Fort I osteotomy with advancement, clockwise maxillary occlusal plane rotation with posterior superior repositioning and anterior vertical lengthening, and a balancing genioplasty (*C, D*).

A   **B**

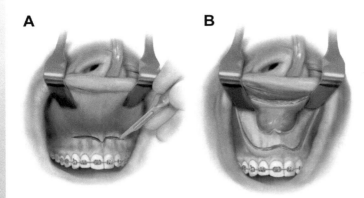

Fig. 6. In patients who have undergone prior midface distraction, the pedicle to the Le Fort I segment can be maximized by maintaining a short incision (*A*), from canine to canine (or first premolar if the lateral incisor is missing). This approach reliably affords access to the pertinent anatomic landmarks for the Le Fort I osteotomy: the infraorbital nerves, piriform rims, and zygomatico-maxillary buttresses (*B*). (*From* Susarla SM, Ettinger RE, Egbert MA. Transmucosal Pterygomaxillary Separation in the Le Fort I Osteotomy. Plast Reconstr Surg. 2020 May;145(5):1262-1265.)

A   **B**

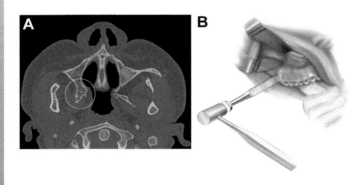

Fig. 7. Following midface distraction, the bony generate is typically formed in the pterygomaxillary junctions (*A, yellow circle*). This can make the pterygomaxillary separation challenging. Using a transmucosal approach through the tuberosity (*B*) can be advantageous in this context, as the surgeon does not need to maneuver a large osteotome through the mucosal pocket, the trajectory of the osteotome can be more easily controlled and monitored, and the bone is often less dense. (*From* Susarla SM, Ettinger RE, Egbert MA. Transmucosal Pterygomaxillary Separation in the Le Fort I Osteotomy. Plast Reconstr Surg. 2020 May;145(5):1262-1265.)

A   **B**

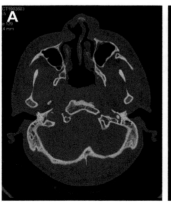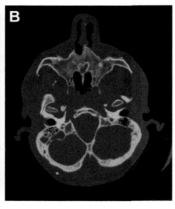

Fig. 8. The maxillary sinus anatomy may be significantly altered by subcranial distraction. In some patients, the maxillary sinuses will be attenuated (*A*). In others, there may be no significant sinus development (*B*). The surgeon must be keenly aware of these variations in anatomy in the context of performing the anterior maxillary osteotomy.

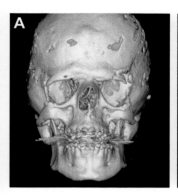
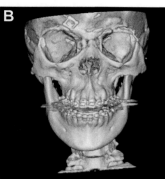

Fig. 9. Patients with syndromic synostosis frequently present with altered piriform anatomy ((A) Crouzon syndrome with history of Le Fort III distraction, (B) Apert syndrome with history of Le Fort II distraction). The piriform rim may be well above the posterior nasal floor. If the anterior maxillary osteotomy cut is placed relative to the native piriform rim, this may be unfavorably high and create challenges navigating around the infraorbital nerve and a posterior osteotomy that is close to the orbital floor. In these situations, surgically lowering the piriform rim using a pear-shaped bur will facilitate placing the osteotomy lower, as well as affording the advantage of expanding the internal nasal valve.

operated midface. Special care should be exercised to maintain perfusion in these cases. Treatment planning in these patients should take into consideration the presence of previously repaired cleft palate or alveolar ridge augmentation.

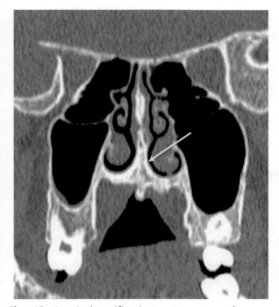

Fig. 10. Atypical ossification patterns can be seen following subcranial midface advancement. In this patient, there is a significant thickening of the vomer at the maxillary crest (arrow, 5–7 mm medio-lateral width). Successful separation of the maxilla from the vomer may require the use of piezoelectric or oscillating saws. When encountering this morphology, the surgeon should consider performing the septal osteotomy after the anterior maxillary, pterygomaxillary, and lateral nasal osteotomies are completed. This will allow for some inferior mobilization of the maxilla and improved visualization of the posterior maxillary crest.

Specific challenges related to prior midface distraction should be considered when considering Le Fort I osteotomies (Figs. 6–11). Technical modifications are primarily related to incision design, pterygomaxillary separation, anticipation of altered maxillary sinus and nasal anatomy, and posterior soft tissue release to allow full mobilization of the Le Fort I segment.

Incisions - Incision planning will need to account for the placement of prior intraoral incisions for Le Fort II or Le Fort III osteotomies. It is our preference to use a narrow mucosal incision (see Fig. 6), extending no further posterior than the distal aspects of the canines (or first premolars in patients missing lateral incisors), to allow for a broad soft tissue pedicle to the Le Fort I segment.

Pterygomaxillary separation - The generate formed following subcranial distraction may be most robust in the pterygomaxillary region.[25] The pterygomaxillary separation in these patients may be challenging due to thick bone within the junction. Our practice is to perform the pterygomaxillary separation transmucosally through the tuberosity (see Fig. 7).[26] We feel that this approach affords several advantages: (1) the bone of the tuberosity tends to be thinner, (2) the osteotome can be directed slightly superiorly without concern for inadvertent penetration into the orbit, and (3) the risk of buccal mucosal tear is greatly reduced, as one does not need to maneuver a sizable osteotome into the pterygomaxillary junction through the mucoperiosteal pocket.

Altered maxillary sinus anatomy – Following subcranial midface advancement, pneumatization of the maxillary sinuses will be inconsistent (see Fig. 8). In some patients, the sinuses are present but diminutive; in others, the sinuses may be

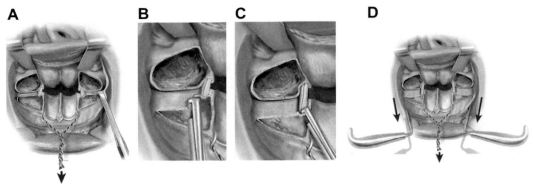

Fig. 11. Following downfracture, the maxilla will need to be fully mobilized to passively sit in the final position. Patients who have undergone prior subcranial distraction will frequently have excess bone and soft tissue scar along the posterior and posterolateral maxilla. Once the maxilla is downfractured, the soft tissue tether can be bluntly released using a periosteal elevator (*A*), followed by iterative bony removal of the posterior maxillary wall (*B*), including ostectomy around the descending palatine neurovascular bundle (*C*). Anterior traction using piriform wires, combined with posterior traction with pterygoid lifts (*D*) will allow for maximum mobilization of the maxilla and passive placement into the final position.

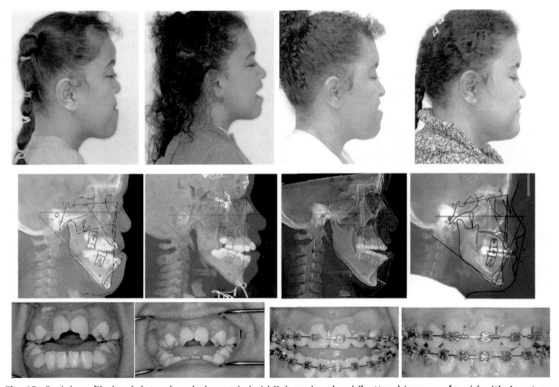

Fig. 12. Facial profile (top), lateral cephalometric (middle), and occlusal (bottom) images of a girl with Apert syndrome are shown. In the early mixed dentition (left images), this patient had nasomaxillary hypoplasia > orbitozygomatic hypoplasia. The midface position was notably improved following Le Fort II + ZR (middle left). At skeletal maturity (middle right), the patient had an end-stage discrepancy characterized by maxillary sagittal hypoplasia, posterior vertical maxillary excess, and asymmetric mandibular prognathism, with a large anterior open bite. She underwent bimaxillary orthognathic surgery and genioplasty (right) with improvement in her occlusion and facial form.

completely absent. When performing the anterior maxillary osteotomy, the surgeon needs to be cognizant of the bony thickness to ensure that the cortical cut is complete, to avoid creating a stress-riser effect when attempting to down fracture the Le Fort I segment.

Altered nasal cavity anatomy – Alterations in nasal cavity anatomy may result in a narrow nasal aperture, superiorly located piriform rim, and unpredictable ossification of the vomer-palatine junction. In these patients, placement of the Le Fort I anterior maxillary osteotomy cut above the level of the piriform may result in an osteotomy that is higher than desired (see **Fig. 9**). The surgeon may elect to lower the piriform rim in these patients, to facilitate more inferior placement of the anterior maxillary osteotomy cut. Doing so carries the additional advantage of expanding the internal nasal valve, the inferior extent of which is defined by the piriform margin.

In some instances, generate from subcranial distraction can be seen at the junction of the vomer with the hard palate, which may make the septal osteotomy challenging (see **Fig. 10**). In these situations, the surgeon may choose to complete the nasal septal osteotomy as the last in the sequence of osteotomies before down fracture. This will enable more direct visualization of the junction of the vomer with the maxillary crest/palate, as the anterior maxilla will be somewhat mobile and able to be retracted inferiorly. Separation of the bony fusion here can then be reliably accomplished under direct visualization with osteotomes or piezoelectric/oscillating saws, with a finger placed over the posterior nasal spine to protect the endotracheal tube and verify separation.

Soft tissue release – Following down fracture, full mobilization of the maxilla is necessary to achieve passive positioning and reduce the risk of relapse. In many patients following subcranial midface distraction, there is abundant soft tissue scarring along the posterior and posterolateral walls of the maxilla. In these situations, meticulous release of the periosteum/scar along the posterior aspect of the maxilla, similar to technical modifications used in the cleft Le Fort I osteotomy, including ostectomy around the descending palatine vessels, with synchronous gentle traction anteriorly (eg, using piriform wires) and posteriorly

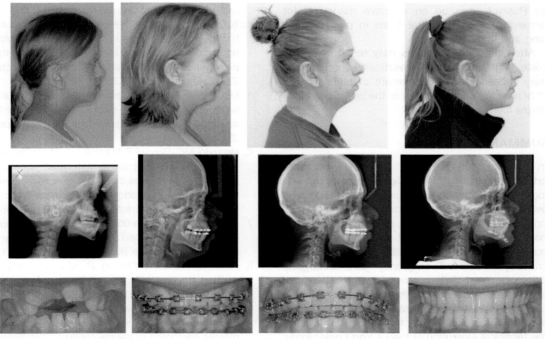

Fig. 13. Facial profile (top), lateral cephalometric (middle), and occlusal (bottom) images of a girl with Crouzon syndrome are shown. In the early mixed dentition (left images), this patient had nasomaxillary hypoplasia = orbitozygomatic hypoplasia. The midface position was notably improved following Le Fort III distraction (middle left). At skeletal maturity (middle right), the patient had an end-stage discrepancy characterized by bimaxillary retrognathism. She underwent bimaxillary orthognathic surgery and genioplasty (right) with improvement in her occlusion and facial form.

(eg, using pterygoid lifts) results in reliable mobilization of the maxilla (see **Fig. 11**).[27]

Mandibular surgery: As stated previously, the mandible in patients with syndromic synostosis ranges from normal in length to having a longer ramus height and a shorter body. The decision to operate on the mandible depends on the presence of mandibular and maxillary asymmetry, facial esthetics, and history of obstructive sleep apnea. Counterclockwise rotational movements of the mandible appear to be stable with appropriate rigid fixation, particularly in patients with normal temporomandibular joints, and can be used to close anterior open bites; however, nearly all patients will require concomitant maxillary surgery to address the primary morphologic deficiencies in the lower midface.

When performing sagittal split ramus osteotomies in this population, the surgeon needs to consider the specific morphologic differences that may be present. Patients with long ramus heights may have mandibular foramina that are located high and posterior or obscured by thick internal oblique ridges. In these patients, ostectomy of the internal oblique ridge may be required to visualize the entry point of the inferior alveolar nerve into the mandible. Alternatively, the low and short medial osteotomy cut, as popularized by Posnick, can be an effective maneuver for achieving reliable sagittal splits in patients with long and thin rami.[28,29]

Attenuated body heights may result in buccal plate segments that are vertically short, which may necessitate the placement of plate fixation at or near the inferior border or the use of bicortical screw fixation.

SUMMARY/DISCUSSION

In patients with a history of craniosynostosis, orthognathic surgery is an effective tool for managing the end-stage skeletal discrepancy.[28] Focused evaluation of the facial morphology as well as concomitant morbidities (eg, obstructive sleep apnea) is essential to arrive at an appropriate diagnosis and surgical plan. Patients with syndromic craniosynostosis will frequently have undergone prior subcranial midface advancement. In this population, one must consider the specific morphologic consequences of subcranial distraction on the morphology of the maxilla that will, in turn, affect the technical execution of the Le Fort I osteotomy. With a coordinated orthodontic-surgical approach, the end-stage skeletal malocclusion that is seen in patients with craniosynostosis can be successfully managed with maxillary and mandibular osteotomies (**Figs. 12** and **13**).

CLINICS CARE POINTS

- Patients with syndromic craniosynostosis undergoing orthognathic evaluation should have a focused assessment of sleep-disordered breathing.
- Following orthognathic surgery, consideration should be given for ICU care in patients with complex airway anatomy, though most patients can be managed in non-ICU settings with appropriate monitoring (eg, continuous pulse oximetry).

REFERENCES

1. Kimonis V, Gold JA, Hoffman TL, et al. Genetics of craniosynostosis. Semin Pediatr Neurol 2007;14:150.
2. Forrest CR, Hopper RA. Craniofacial syndromes and surgery. Plast Reconstr Surg 2012;131:86e.
3. Posnick JC, Ruiz RL. The craniofacial dysostosis syndromes: current surgical thinking and future directions. Cleft Palate Craniofac J 2000;37:433.
4. Burdi AR, Kusnetz AB, Venes JL, et al. The natural history and pathogenesis of the cranial coronal ring articulations: implications in understanding the pathogenesis of the Crouzon craniostenotic defects. Cleft Palate J 1986;23(1):28–39.
5. McGrath J, Gerety PA, Derderian CA, et al. Differential closure of the spheno-occipital synchondrosis in syndromic craniosynostosis. Plast Reconstr Surg 2012;130(5):681e–9e.
6. Meazzini MC, Corradi F, Mazzoleni F, et al. Circummaxillary sutures in patients with apert, crouzon, and pfeiffer syndromes compared to nonsyndromic children: growth, orthodontic, and surgical implications. Cleft Palate Craniofac J 2021;58(3):299–305.
7. Watts GD, Antonarakis GS, Blaser SI, et al. Craniorbital morphology caused by coronal ring suture synostosis. Plast Reconstr Surg 2019;144(6):1403–11.
8. Forte AJ, Alonso N, Persing JA, et al. Analysis of midface retrusion in Crouzon and Apert syndromes. Plast Reconstr Surg 2014;134(2):285–93.
9. Reitsma JH, Ongkosuwito EM, Buschang PH, et al. Facial growth in patients with apert and crouzon syndromes compared to normal children. Cleft Palate Craniofac J 2012;49(2):185–93.
10. Zhou X, Pu D, Liu R, et al. The Fgfr2(S252W/+) mutation in mice retards mandible formation and reduces bone mass as in human Apert syndrome. Am J Med Genet A 2013;161A(5):983–92.

11. Kreiborg S. Crouzon Syndrome. A clinical and roentgencephalometric study. Scand J Plast Reconstr Surg Suppl 1981;18:1–198.

12. Costaras-Volarich M, Pruzansky S. Is the mandible intrinsically different in Apert and Crouzon syndromes? Am J Orthod 1984;85(6):475–87.

13. Wink JD, Bastidas N, Bartlett SP. Analysis of the long-term growth of the mandible in Apert syndrome. J Craniofac Surg 2013;24(4):1408–10.

14. Reitsma JH, Elmi P, Ongkosuwito EM, et al. A longitudinal study of dental arch morphology in children with the syndrome of Crouzon or Apert. Eur J Oral Sci 2013;121(4):319–27.

15. Agochukwu NB, Solomon BD, Doherty ES, et al. Palatal and oral manifestations of Muenke syndrome (FGFR3-related craniosynostosis). J Craniofac Surg 2012;23(3):664–8.

16. Hopper RA, Kapadia H, Susarla SM. Surgical-orthodontic considerations in subcranial and frontofacial distraction. Oral Maxillofac Surg Clin North Am 2020;32(2):309–20.

17. Liu MT, Kurnik NM, Mercan E, et al. Magnitude of horizontal advancement is associated with apnea hypopnea index improvement and counterclockwise maxillary rotation after subcranial distraction for syndromic synostosis. J Oral Maxillofac Surg 2021;79(5):1133.e1–16.

18. Hopper RA, Wang HD, Mercan E. Le Fort II distraction with simultaneous zygomatic repositioning. Clin Plast Surg 2021;48(3):487–96.

19. Taylor JA, Bartlett SP. What's New in Syndromic Craniosynostosis Surgery? Plast Reconstr Surg 2017;140(1):82e–93e.

20. Hopper RA, Kapadia H, Susarla SM. Le Fort II distraction with zygomatic repositioning: a technique for differential correction of midface hypoplasia. J Oral Maxillofac Surg 2018;76(9):2002.e1–14.

21. Allareddy V. Orthognathic surgeries in patients with congenital craniofacial anomalies: profile and hospitalization outcomes. Cleft Palate Craniofac J 2015;52(6):698–705.

22. Ferri J, Schlund M, Touzet-Roumazeille S. Orthognathic Surgery in Craniosynostosis. J Craniofac Surg 2021;32(1):141–8.

23. Chow LK, Singh B, Chiu WK, et al. Prevalence of postoperative complications after orthognathic surgery: a 15-year review. J Oral Maxillofac Surg 2007;65(5):984–92.

24. Resnick CM, Kim S, Yorlets RR, et al. Evaluation of Andrews' analysis as a predictor of ideal sagittal maxillary positioning in orthognathic surgery. J Oral Maxillofac Surg 2018;76(10):2169–76.

25. Hopper RA, Sandercoe G, Woo A, et al. Computed tomographic analysis of temporal maxillary stability and pterygomaxillary generate formation following pediatric Le Fort III distraction advancement. Plast Reconstr Surg 2010;126(5):1665–74.

26. Susarla SM, Ettinger RE, Egbert MA. Transmucosal pterygomaxillary separation in the Le Fort I osteotomy. Plast Reconstr Surg 2020;145(5):1262–5.

27. Susarla SM, Ettinger R, Preston K, et al. Technical modifications specific to the Cleft Le Fort I Osteotomy. J Craniofac Surg 2020;31(5):1459–63.

28. Posnick JC, Choi E, Liu S. Occurrence of a 'bad' split and success of initial mandibular healing: a review of 524 sagittal ramus osteotomies in 262 patients. Int J Oral Maxillofac Surg 2016;45(10):1187–94.

29. Susarla SM, Cho DY, Ettinger RE, et al. The Low medial horizontal osteotomy in patients with atypical ramus morphology undergoing sagittal split osteotomy. J Oral Maxillofac Surg 2020;78(10):1813–9.